SHOT

SHOT
Staying Alive with Diabetes

Amy F. Ryan

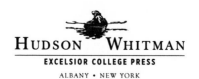

HUDSON WHITMAN
EXCELSIOR COLLEGE PRESS
ALBANY • NEW YORK

This is a work of nonfiction. However, some names and
identifying details have been changed to protect the privacy of individuals.

This book is not intended as a substitute for the medical advice of physicians.
The reader should regularly consult a physician in matters relating
to his/her health and particularly with respect to any symptoms
that may require diagnosis or medical attention.

Published by Hudson Whitman/Excelsior College Press
7 Columbia Circle, Albany, NY 12203
www.hudsonwhitman.com

Printed in the United States of America
Book design by Melissa Mykal Batalin
Cover design by Phil Pascuzzo

LCCN: 2012950669

ISBN: 978-0-9768813-5-3

First Edition

To everyone who understands this story
because it is part of their own.

PART I

1

My 29th year was off to a great start. I had been promoted at work. I'd been accepted in one of the top law schools in the country. I'd lost some weight. I was dating a man who had two little boys, and I adored all three of them. Then I got a yeast infection.

A yeast infection sounded harmless enough. I'd never had one before, but my doctor assured me it was a common condition suffered by many women.

"Are you sexually active?" she asked.

"Yep."

"Same guy as before? Still monogamous?"

"Yes and yes."

"Still going to the gym regularly?"

"Yep."

"It's probably some combination of all of those. Be sure to use the bathroom after sex, don't keep on damp exercise clothes after your workout, and be sure to wear cotton underpants."

She gave me a prescription for a medication to be administered every night when I went to bed for the next several nights, and she cautioned me to wear cotton underwear and to keep dry. "And, by the way," she mentioned just before slipping out of the examination room, "there was some sugar in your urine. You might want to have that checked the next time you see your GP."

"Checked for what?" I asked.

"Diabetes," she said casually. "You're an unlikely candidate, but the sugar in your urine was high. So you should have it checked at some point." She paused for a moment while looking at my chart and then asked, "Did you eat breakfast before you came in today?"

"Yes."

"What did you eat?"

Sheepishly, I responded, "Honey Nut Cheerios." Paul, the man whom I was dating, often teased me for having the culinary preferences of a twelve-year-old, so it was with some embarrassment that I made this admission to my doctor.

"That's probably it. It's probably just all that sugar from the cereal getting out of your system." She closed her chart and looked up at me, saying, "Take care." And she was gone.

Diabetes. I would have to remember to get that checked. But not before I went away for a long weekend with Paul. We had rented an oceanfront condominium for Memorial Day weekend, a little more than a week away. That gave me just enough time to finish the prescription for my yeast infection and be in good shape for our vacation.

I took the last dose of my prescription on a Monday night. By Wednesday, all of the symptoms had returned. *Strange*, I thought. *I must have somehow screwed up the medicine.*

I called my gynecologist's office first thing Thursday morning. I needed to get this cleared up as soon as possible. A weekend at the beach treating a yeast infection was not what I had in mind.

"Dr. Anderson doesn't have any appointments open," the receptionist informed me when I asked whether my doctor could see me that day.

"I'm not trying to be a pain. It's just that I leave on Saturday for vacation, and I really need to see her before then. How about if I just come in and wait, and whoever is available first can see me?"

"Well, you can try that," she replied. "We open at eight. If you're here at eight, someone can probably see you."

I got ready for work in half the time it usually took and rushed across town so that I could be at the doctor's office when the door opened. As I drove, I chuckled to myself as I imagined how impressed

Paul would have been that I was presentable and downtown by 8:00 a.m. He was decidedly a morning person, and I was decidedly not. My inability to function before 9:00 was a constant source of amusement for him. Paul was out of town for a three-day conference in New York and was due back the following day, Friday. Saturday morning we were leaving for the beach. Although I missed him disproportionately when he was gone, I was glad he was not in town to endure my "female issue." He would have had as little interest in hearing about it as I had in sharing the information with him, and so I wasn't disappointed to deal with the recurrence by myself.

I arrived at my doctor's office just as the doors were being unlocked.

"Hi, I'm Amy Fitzgerald," I said as I approached the reception desk. "I called just a while ago. Did I talk to you?"

"You did. I told one of our nurse midwives, Connie, that you were coming in. If you just go on back to Room 4, Connie will be right in."

A nurse midwife. Interesting. I was not pregnant, of course, but if a nurse midwife was available, then a nurse midwife it would be. I had never met Connie. In my several years as a patient of that practice, I had dealt primarily with my doctor, Dr. Anderson, the one who the week earlier had advised me to have my blood sugar level checked by my GP. I was lucky enough to have found a physician who took an individual interest in each of her patients, who personally returned telephone calls the very same day, and who did not send a nurse to do the doctor's job.

Connie entered the exam room, closing the door behind her. "What's going on with you?"

"Well, I just finished a prescription for a yeast infection two days ago, and right away my symptoms came back. I'm about to go on vacation, and I really want to get this cleared up."

"I'm sure you do," Connie replied sympathetically. "Here's what we need to do. I need to get your weight. And then, if you would, just pop across the hall into the bathroom and give me a urine specimen. Come back in here, change into this robe, and I will be right back in to do a culture. We'll have you out of here in no time. Now, take your shoes off and step up on the scale."

I did as instructed.

"One hundred sixteen pounds," Connie recited.

"Really?" I asked, surprised. "What was I at my last appointment? I'm usually closer to 130."

"Let me see," Connie said as she leafed through my file. "You're right. You weighed 132 pounds at your annual exam just five months ago. Have you been dieting? Doing anything differently?"

"No, I'm doing everything the same as usual. I haven't changed a thing."

"Hmmm. I'll note that weight loss here in your file. Now if you can just go and give me that urine sample."

Again I did as instructed. I marked the clear specimen cup with my name, gave the specimen, and placed it on the designated shelf in the bathroom for a lab technician to collect. Then I went back into the exam room and changed into the papery robe that Connie had left for me.

Connie knocked and re-entered the room. "You have a lot of sugar in your urine," she told me. "Has that happened before?"

"No one had ever mentioned it before, but when I came in for the yeast infection last week, the doctor told me the same thing. Should I be worried about that?"

"We'll see," she said. She had me lie down on the table and put my feet in the stirrups, and then she swabbed me for a culture. "That's all. Let me take this out to the lab, and you can change back into your clothes. I'll be back in just a few minutes."

I did as instructed and waited for Connie to return.

"Wow" was her first word when she returned to the exam room. "You have so much yeast, it just jumped off the slide. So that's what it is—another yeast infection."

"Why another one? I just finished my treatment."

"I'm not sure, but I am concerned about the sugar in your urine. That's probably what's causing the infections—yeast thrives in a sugary environment. I want to do another test, just a finger stick, to see what the glucose level is in your blood."

A finger stick. Ugh. I didn't like being stuck, and I didn't like blood. But I would endure anything if I could just get better in time for my vacation.

Connie left the room and returned a few minutes later with a small machine about the size of a deck of cards. She pushed the power button to turn it on and then inserted a small strip. "I'm just going to squeeze your finger and prick it to get a drop of blood. You'll feel a little sting, but that's all." Connie did just what she had described, and squeezed a drop of my blood onto the strip that was inserted into the machine. The machine beeped when my blood came in contact with the strip. It beeped again about 20 seconds later, and a number appeared on the display screen.

"Three hundred twenty-three," she said. "Oh, gosh, that's high."

"What does it mean?" I asked, unaware as yet of the dizzying world of blood glucose levels that would soon dominate my life.

"It means that you have diabetes," was her stark reply.

I was stunned. I struggled to comprehend what she had said. "Could it mean anything else?" I stammered. "Is there anything else that could make me have that number?" I didn't know what that number meant. I knew only that Connie was noticeably worried. "What's a normal number?" It was so hard to think of the right questions to ask.

"A normal number is in the 90s—323 is definitely not normal. There's really nothing other than diabetes that would cause your glucose level to be so high. That's why you're having the yeast infections."

Oh, God. This sounded serious. My heart was racing. I struggled to swallow. Connie sensed my distress. "Here's what you need to do. You need to call your GP and tell him that you just had a glucose test, and your blood glucose level is 323. Your GP will take it from there. He'll probably refer you to an endocrinologist."

"But what does this mean? Am I going to be okay?"

"Just call your GP. Call today. Call as soon as you can." And with that, Connie hugged me. "Don't worry. You're going to be okay."

A hug from a nurse midwife, as comforting as it may be, could not be a good sign. They hug people they want to shelter from a world they are about to enter. They hug people who at that moment have nothing else to cling to, literally or figuratively. I sensed all that. I knew Connie was genuinely sorry that I was about to go through something she wished I didn't have to endure. As desperate as it made me feel, I was grateful for the hug.

I toyed with the idea of going home to make the call to my general practitioner. But it was my last day in the office before the long weekend, and I had a few loose ends to tie up. I drove the fifteen minutes to work, thinking there must be some explanation other than what Connie had told me.

I called my general practitioner's office shortly after I arrived at work and settled in at my cubicle. My cubicle was "semi-private." "Private" meant that my co-workers could not see me, but the "semi" meant that they could hear me. We all had partitions around our desks, the walls of which extended to a point several feet shy of the ceiling. I chose my words carefully, knowing they were all being overheard.

In a semi-hushed voice, I said to the receptionist who answered the phone, "I need to leave a message for a doctor or nurse. I just had a blood glucose test at my gyne..." No, I wasn't going to say "gynecologist" in earshot of my co-workers. "I just had a blood glucose test, and I was told I should call the doctor right away with the results." The receptionist took down my name and phone number and said she would deliver my message to one of the nurses.

Feeling satisfied that I had fulfilled my obligation and hoping that no one would call me back before I left for my long weekend, I began to organize my tasks for the day. If I could just impose some order, perhaps I could get back on track. No sooner had I assembled my daily list of things to do, though, than the phone rang. The nurse from my doctor's office was on the line. "Miss Fitzgerald? I got your message. Is there an issue with your blood sugar?"

"I'm really not sure," I began. "I just came from an appointment at my gynecologist's off—" *Damn.* "She said that I had a high level of sugar in my urine. And she did this finger-prick test and told me a number that I should tell the doctor is my glucose level."

"What was the number?" the nurse asked calmly.

"Three hundred twenty-three," I said.

"DID YOU SAY 323? OH, MY GOD," she exclaimed. "How far along are you?"

"How far along am I?" I asked, utterly confused.

"How many months pregnant are you?"

"Pregnant? I'm not pregnant." I could smell the sizzle from the semi-private ears burning all around my cubicle—*Amy Fitzgerald saw a gynecologist, had a urine test, and she said the word "pregnant" during a call with the doctor's office.*

"Oh, thank God," sighed the nurse. Then, after a pause, she continued, "You need to come in. Today. How soon can you be here?"

"Twenty minutes."

"Come on in. We'll be waiting for you."

I left my office immediately and drove to my second doctor's office of the day. It wasn't hot. It was searing. I drove without the air conditioner, with the windows open, hoping that the oppressive heat would give me something to think about other than how the nurse had reacted to my number. It almost worked.

Arriving at the doctor's office, I was hustled through reception as if I were in fact pregnant and my water had just broken. I was whisked away to an examination room immediately.

"Amy," the nurse who was assigned to me said gently. Never had I heard my name delivered so pitifully. "How are you feeling?"

"Fine, I think. A little worried, I guess, about this glucose thing."

"Let me ask you a few questions about that," the nurse said calmly. It was clear that she was taking great pains not to overtax me. "Have you been very thirsty lately?"

"I don't know. I'm a drinker. I'm always drinking something. I drink a liter of water a day. I drink Diet Coke. I drink beer. I don't notice being thirsty, but maybe that's because I'm always drinking something." Hearing myself say all that, it sounded as though I were making excuses rather than answering the question. This wasn't the time for a chicken-or-egg debate about my thirst.

"Do you urinate frequently?" asked the nurse.

"I do. But, as I said, I drink a lot. So I pee a lot." As I said that, I recalled a recent conversation with Paul. We had played our weekly racquetball match and then had gone out for our traditional cheeseburger and beers afterwards. Back at my apartment after dinner, I had to excuse myself several times within a short time period to use the bathroom.

"I've never seen anybody use the bathroom as often as you do," Paul had said.

"Oh, I'm sure it's just the beer," I replied.

"Well, I drank beer, too, and I'm not using the bathroom every fifteen minutes." Then, after a pause, he said, "Maybe you have some kind of a condition."

"What do you mean, 'a condition?'" I had asked. "What kind of condition makes you have to pee all the time?" Oh, ignorance is indeed bliss.

Recalling this conversation, whose relevance now was becoming apparent, I slipped emotionally just a little. If frequent urination was an issue, I was a goner. Regardless of how much I drank in a given day, remembering that conversation with Paul was a red alert: In the opinion of a man who could find no fault with me, I peed a lot.

"Yes, you could say I urinate frequently," I said slowly to the nurse.

"Do you have blurry vision?" she continued.

"No, my vision is perfect."

"Have you lost weight recently?" That one took the wind out of my sails.

Before I answered, I recalled my weight as Connie had recited it earlier that day: 116 pounds, down from 132 five months earlier. I also recalled, in the same hazy manner that I had recalled my conversation with Paul, one of the trainers at my gym asking me a few weeks earlier if I had lost weight. "I don't think so," I had responded. I never weighed myself. My clothes still fit me, even if they sagged a little, but I was strong and in great shape. "Just checking," he responded. "You look to me like you're wasting away. I want to make sure you're taking care of yourself." Then I remembered, around the same time, that a particularly unsocial co-worker had gone out of her way to ask me if I was all right. "I don't want to pry," she had said, "but is everything okay? You're so skinny lately, and you look so tired."

"Amy?" the nurse asked, summoning me back. "Have you been losing weight lately?"

"Umm, yes. Yes, I have," I mumbled, the questions and answers beginning to ricochet in my head. *This number of 323, plus the fact that I drink all the time, plus the fact that I pee more than anyone Paul has ever met, plus my recent weight loss, all seem to be pointing toward a serious diagnosis of some sort.*

"Okay, I need you to go into that bathroom across the hall and give me a urine sample. Be sure and follow the instructions posted in the bathroom about writing your name on the cup."

I didn't respond. I just did as I was told. I walked across the hall slowly, deliberately, making sure before each step that the floor was solid beneath me. I didn't feel as if I could be sure of anything at that point. I closed the door to the bathroom. I marked my name on the cup. I pulled up my skirt and pulled down my underpants. I wiped myself as instructed in the directions posted on the wall. I peed into the cup. I placed the cup into the two-way cabinet, just as I had earlier that morning.

I refastened my skirt, washed my hands, and cracked open the bathroom door. I heard a report being passed along among the staff. The voices that I overheard were lowered. I knew right away they were talking about me. "She's spilling ketones...major ketones in her urine...probably heading toward ketoacidosis...." Whatever ketones were, and whatever this other keto-acid-something-or-other word was, none of it sounded very good. The tone of the voices was grave. It was a tone far more serious than anyone wants to hear in a doctor's office with reference to her own health.

I returned to the exam room, and the nurse entered right behind me and closed the door. "Amy," she began earnestly, with another heart-wrenching rendition of my name, "we're sending you to an endocrinologist. We're referring you to a doctor who is just about ten minutes away from here. We're getting the paperwork ready now. Is there anyone you can call? Someone who could drive you from here to the endocrinologist's office?"

"I have a car here. I don't need anyone to drive me." What was she talking about? Had she confused me with some other patient?

"I'm not sure whether it's safe for you to drive," she said.

"Why wouldn't it be safe?"

"You have a very high level of ketones in your urine. You could be going into a coma," she responded somberly. Then, after a short pause she added, "But let me check about that."

Yes, could you, please? I thought to myself. *Perhaps you could have checked about that before you mentioned it?* And what did she mean—a coma? I had heard of a diabetic coma, and it didn't take an endocrinologist to infer that a diabetic coma must be what she was talking about. But how did it happen? Could I be driving to the next doctor's office and suddenly lose consciousness when, right now, other than being completely panicked, I felt pretty much okay?

The nurse slipped out into the hall to inquire as to my likely state of consciousness for the next few minutes. I heard her ask someone, "Do you think Miss Fitzgerald is fine to drive to the endocrinologist's office?"

"Sure, he's only ten minutes away," a male voice responded.

The nurse re-entered my exam room, appearing to be much relieved. "Amy," she said in a more lighthearted tone, "you're fine to drive. Stop by the referral desk on the way out, pick up your paperwork for the other doctor, and then go straight to his office. Good luck."

"I have one quick question," I said, gathering up my purse and looking for my car keys. I knew I was barking up the wrong tree, but I had to ask. More importantly, I needed to ask someone who was so woefully uninformed about my condition that she would possibly give me the answer I wanted to hear. "Can I still go to the beach tomorrow?"

"Well, I don't see why not. But you should ask the endocrinologist for sure." Great. If she had said I could go, then surely it wasn't a good idea. Four minutes ago she had me headed for a coma, and now it was okay for me to go the beach? Doubtful. I added the beach question to my mental list of questions to ask the next doctor I would see. The beach question was first. The other questions I hoped could wait until after the long weekend.

I drove directly to the endocrinologist's office, my third doctor's office in about as many hours. Arriving at the office, I was greeted by what I dreaded seeing in the waiting room: sick people. Before that day, I don't think I had noticed much whether the people in waiting rooms were sick or well. I had grown up around sick people. My mother was a nurse at a university hospital. My father, brother, sister, and I would eat dinner with her in the hospital cafeteria when she was working an evening shift. It wasn't unusual for a patient with a tracheotomy to stop by our table and wheeze out his gratitude to my mother, the puckered hole in his neck trying to close itself as he struggled to speak, while we ate our Salisbury steak dinner. So sick people were nothing new for me.

But now, when I saw the sick people in that waiting room, it was in a different light. It was with the sinking realization that I might be one of them. Outwardly I didn't appear to be unhealthy. That was probably the conclusion that the others in the waiting room reached as I made my way to the reception desk. I felt their eyes assess me as I crossed the room. I wasn't overweight, as several of them were. I had two feet, and not all of them did. I didn't wear glasses, and at least half of them had those. *Clearly, I'll be waiting a while,* I thought to myself. *I'm obviously not as serious a case as any of these people.*

I signed in at the reception desk, and the receptionist greeted me right away. "Miss Fitzgerald, we were expecting you. The doctor will see you now. His office is right at the end of that hall. You can go on back."

I was stunned. The doctor was seeing *me* before any of the other people in the waiting room who were so obviously in need of medical attention? There must be some mistake.

"Before we even get started here," the doctor began affably, "let me just calm your nerves about one thing." *Oh, thank goodness,* I thought to myself. *My other doctor's office must have told him about my upcoming vacation, and he's going to start off by letting me know I can still go to the beach.* I settled back more comfortably into the chair across the desk from him and waited to receive the good news.

"Of course, there are no guarantees," he began, "but in all likelihood you should be able to have children. You should be able to have a healthy pregnancy and have a healthy child. Ever since that movie came out, that's the first question every woman your age who has diabetes wants to know: 'Am I going to be able to have children? Am I going to need a kidney transplant if I have a baby?' Oh, I wish that movie had never come out."

What on earth was he talking about? What movie? And what was this about babies? My head swam.

"I'm sorry," I said, confused. "But I don't know what you're talking about. What movie?"

"*Steel Magnolias.* Don't tell me you haven't seen *Steel Magnolias,*" he responded jovially, as if we were meeting at a cocktail party rather than in his office.

"Of course, I've seen it," I said. I, like most every other woman who has seen the movie, cannot forget Shelby, the main character, announcing her ill-advised pregnancy to her mother, declaring that she would rather have thirty minutes' worth of wonderful than a lifetime worth of nothing special. But that was a movie. Why was he talking about a movie when this was real life? "Why are you talking about the movie?" I asked him.

"Diabetes. Shelby had diabetes," the doctor responded excitedly, his arms extended upwardly in a *eureka* gesture. "That's why she was never supposed to get pregnant in the first place. But it's a different world now. Women with diabetes have babies every day and go on to live very normal lives. Oh, I wish that movie had never come out."

How did I not know that Shelby had diabetes? I knew she wasn't supposed to get pregnant, and I knew she ended up with kidney disease, but I must have been out of the room when the other diabetes clues were revealed. *Perhaps I had excused myself to go to the bathroom and pee, as I so often had to do,* I thought ruefully.

I needed some time to regroup. In the space of just a few hours I had been told that I had diabetes (although I still had no idea what that meant) that I could go into a coma, and now a serious question about my ability to have children had been raised. The doctor, observing my utter confusion, transitioned quickly from the role of movie critic to the role of endocrinologist.

"You don't really fit the mold of Type 2, but if I had to guess, I would say that you are not going to need insulin," the doctor informed me after I had debriefed him on my medical history and he had given me the short primer on the two different types of diabetes. He explained that the profile of a typical adult with Type 2 diabetes, also called "adult onset" diabetes, was someone who is overweight, sedentary, and has a poor diet. None of these was me. Still, according to the doctor, it would be odd for a case of Type 1 or "juvenile" diabetes to present itself four months before my 30th birthday. Odd, he said, but certainly not unprecedented. He would try a pill on me first.

"Get this prescription filled today and get started on that. You also need to get a glucose monitor and test your glucose levels four times a day—once before each meal, and once at bedtime. Write down your numbers in a log that I'll give you, and be sure to bring the log back in for your next appointment. I want to see you at the beginning of next week." Handing the glucose log and several pamphlets to me, he added, "And you should read these. They'll answer a lot of questions you probably have."

Before I left, I had to ask the question that I had gone there wanting to have answered. I was pretty sure I knew the answer, but I needed to hear him say it. "Doctor," I began hesitantly, "my boyfriend and I were planning to go to the beach for the long weekend. Can I still go away?"

He looked at me apologetically. "I don't think you should go. We need to get this under control before you think about leaving town."

Honestly, could this be so serious that I couldn't leave town? I'd never left a doctor's office with anything but an antidote for what ailed me. A cast if a bone was broken. Nasal spray if I had a sinus infection. Antibiotics if I had strep throat. But this guy was sending me away without a real solution. He was sending me away with a theory, and with something to try, and with instructions that I shouldn't leave town. I don't think I'd ever had a follow-up visit with a physician. They just fixed me in one visit. But this guy wanted to see me next week, and it sounded as if there might be more appointments after that.

I'd do what he said. I'd get the glucose meter, I'd do the tests, I'd take the pill, and I'd come back next week. And then he might see that he'd been wrong. He might see that my so-called diabetes had cleared up. Maybe all I needed was a little time. Maybe all these doctors didn't know what they were talking about. I just didn't think there was any way they could be right.

2

When I was first diagnosed, in 1996, diabetes wasn't so much in the news. I had heard of it, certainly. My grandmother had diabetes, I knew that, but I didn't really know what it meant. I thought it had something to do with her eating too many sweets. I had also seen a public service poster about diabetes in the locker room of my health club. It listed a few symptoms, advising a few things to be on the watch for. But that didn't have anything to do with me. I wasn't a big sweets eater. I was healthy. I didn't need to read about diabetes.

If I wanted deeper information, I would have had to do some digging—go to a library and ask for help researching diabetes, or find some medical journals. There wasn't a lot of plain talk about the disease, not a lot of information for someone newly diagnosed. Back then I relied on a pamphlet from the American Diabetes Association. I read some words on glossy paper, with images of fruits and vegetables in the background. I saw healthy-looking people riding bicycles, their helmets securely fastened. I stopped briefly at the image of a young woman pricking her finger and smiling gratefully, happy to be living in, apparently, a new era of diabetes technology. There were a few scary parts: here a bullet for heart disease, there a bullet for vision problems. But there was no overwhelming barrage of numbers and statistics—the important information fit into a tri-fold color brochure, after all.

Today, with just a few keystrokes, you can find more information than you might ever want to know about the disease. If I can imagine myself on the day of my diagnosis having the Internet at my disposal, I cannot say what my reaction would have been. How would it have unfolded for me with global data at my fingertips? I think the term "information overload" would not have begun to describe it. The term "complete nervous breakdown" might have captured it better.

I probably would have started with the basics: "What is diabetes?" I would have clicked through to the current source of all knowledge—Wikipedia. My other choices would have been plentiful, and would have included the American Diabetes Association, the World Health Organization, the National Institute for Digestive Disorders and Kidney Disease, the Juvenile Diabetes Research Foundation, and so many others. I may have thought, *Wow, there are a lot of major organizations concerned about this disease. Is that good or bad? Why so much interest in diabetes?*

I would have read through the descriptions of the different types of diabetes. I might have read these quickly because, actually, all I would have wanted was to cut to the chase: *What's going to happen to me?* I really would have wanted to know the worst-case scenario—like most patients who leave a doctor's office with a vague new word that suddenly applies to them as they rush home to begin their solitary research.

I would have learned that there are at least three types of diabetes. There is Type 1 diabetes, also known as insulin-dependent diabetes, or juvenile diabetes, in which the body's immune system attacks and destroys the insulin-producing cells of the pancreas. As a result, the pancreas of a person who has Type 1 diabetes does not produce insulin. People who have Type 1 diabetes need to have multiple, daily injections of insulin in order to survive.

I would not yet have known my type, but I would have guessed this was not my kind. I was not a juvenile. I would have learned that about three million people have Type 1 diabetes. That number—three million—would have slowed me down a bit. *That's a lot of people,* I would have thought, simply, to myself. Then I would have read that many, perhaps as many as half of the cases of newly diagnosed Type 1 diabetes, occurs in adults. That fact would have slowed me down even more. *Adults can get this? Then why is it called juvenile diabetes?*

16

Next on the list would be Type 2 diabetes, also known as non-insulin dependent diabetes, or adult-onset diabetes, in which the pancreas either does not produce enough insulin or the insulin that the pancreas does produce is unable to get into the body's cells. This is by far the more predominant form today: Health professionals currently refer to it as an epidemic. *Maybe that's my kind*, I might have thought. I was, after all, an adult. But I didn't fit the usual suspect list. Many people who have Type 2 diabetes have a poor diet, are overweight, and don't get a lot of exercise. That wasn't my profile at all. I was thin, exercised almost daily, and ate pretty well.

As I kept searching to find where I fit in, I would have read that over twenty million people have Type 2 diabetes. That number would have slowed me down, too. Twenty million people is now, and would certainly have been back then, impossible for me to fathom. *What other diseases affect twenty million people?* I would have wondered. *Is anyone doing anything about this? How can all those people have diabetes?* I'll bet I wouldn't have been thinking "we"—how can "we" all have this? I didn't understand then that I was one of those statistics, no matter which type I had.

Perhaps then I would have read about gestational diabetes, which is the only kind I could have ruled out with certainty, because I wasn't pregnant. I would have learned that gestational diabetes occurs in about five percent of all pregnancies, and that although it typically resolves after delivery, as many as half of the women who had it would develop Type 2 diabetes later in life. By that point, my temples might have been pulsing as I wondered who was *not* going to get diabetes. How were all these people—again, not me—living a life that I knew nothing about?

I would have read on, scrolling down the page to the signs and symptoms. I would have done this whether I wanted to or not, because I wouldn't have been able to resist the color diagram of the human body with arrows drawn out from so many different organs and systems, with explanatory legends by each. There's the central nervous system (*that's a biggie*, I would have thought), listing the symptoms of stupor and lethargy. There are the eyes (*certainly a close second to the brain*), with a note indicating blurry vision. Move down just a bit, and there's the windpipe, denoting that the breath may have a chemical smell. And move just a bit further down to the lungs (*also pretty high up on the list of necessary organs*) indicating that the patient may hyperventilate. Next, the stomach, with arrows out for nausea, vomiting, and abdominal pain. And last but not least, the urinary system, indicating frequent urination. I would have been grateful that the model was only from the waist up. Half the body alone was more than I wanted to know.

By that point, the information would have been fairly well jammed into my head—confusing me, scaring me—and I wouldn't have felt that I could take much more. But I would have read on—how could I not? The entry would have been almost twenty pages long. Twenty pages. Almost as long as the entry for the U.S. Constitution. Almost as long as the entry for the Civil War.

I'll bet I would have been barely skimming at that point, unable to process what I was taking in, yet pausing momentarily to absorb each new knot in my gut as I read phrases such as: altered states of consciousness... rare but severe... reduced vision... potential blindness... scarring in the kidney... eventually requiring dialysis... impact on the nervous system... vascular disease... foot ulcers... require amputation.

Never mind that the word "occasionally" appears before the words "require amputation." The word "occasionally" would have done nothing to lessen the blow of reading it for the first time. It does nothing to cushion the blow of reading it for the fiftieth time, for that matter.

Okay, deep breath. I would have taken a deep breath and tried to regroup. Then I might have taken a step back and tried another angle. I might have tried to figure out why this had happened. I would have gone to the "Causes" section of the Wiki entry. I would have found any number of possible causes: genetic defects in beta cell function, genetic defects in insulin processing or insulin action, exocrine pancreatic defects. But these would have been just words. Black marks on a screen. They were technical words, medical words that would have meant nothing to me. Nothing could answer—nothing ever would answer—what I really wanted to know: *Why me?* But before I would have let myself fall too far into self-pity, I might have had just enough gumption left to pull myself back up and try one more thing. I might have realized I had not seen the section in which they talk about the cure for diabetes. I must have missed that. So I would scroll up, and I would scroll down. But there would have been too many pages to cover. I would not have been able to find the section on the cure. So I would have typed the phrase "cure for diabetes" into the search box. And I would have been met, there and then, with the sentence that would stop me cold: There is no cure for diabetes.

NO CURE.

Two more severe words do not exist.

I wouldn't beam up to the no-cure reality for some time. That fact was not highlighted in my tri-fold color brochure. Back in 1996, the main feeling I got from that brochure was that I was part of some new group of people whom I didn't know—the faces on the brochure. They were happy. They were smiling. They were getting glucose readings of 108 on their meters. They were exercising and eating fruit. Who were these glossy-pamphlet people?

I thought I might find some of my kind at the American Diabetes Association. I noticed in one of my brochures that the ADA had its headquarters just a few miles from my apartment in Alexandria, Virginia. I decided to head over there. It was an association, after all. Maybe a bunch of people with diabetes would be hanging around, associating.

Other than a receptionist, the lobby of the ADA was empty and quiet. I introduced myself and told her I was there for information. I'd just been diagnosed, and I was trying to find whatever was available and maybe find out how to meet other people who had diabetes.

The receptionist directed me to a rack of pamphlets, and she pointed out a bulletin board that had information about diabetes support groups in the area. She also handed me a magazine, *Diabetes Forecast*, and said there was a pen-pal section in the back.

I walked over to the bulletin board and looked at some of the support group offerings. They all met at area hospitals during the evening. Did I want to spend an evening at a meeting room in a hospital, sitting around talking to a group of people with diabetes? No. That's not what the people in the brochures did.

I went home and read the magazine. It had good, informative articles and tasty recipes. I flipped to the back and read a few of the pen-pal solicitations. The average one read like this,

> "Adult with Type 1 diabetes. Suffer from depression and have lost interest in many day-to-day activities. Frustrated with trying to control my glucose levels. Eyesight failing. Looking to share experiences with someone who understands. Inmates need not reply."

Whoa. This was not a group I wanted to be a part of.

Though I didn't have the Internet then, and didn't have the wealth of immediate information that may have been more of a curse than a blessing, I also didn't have a community. The faces in the brochures weren't comforting to me. They didn't make me feel like I was a part of anything at all. They made me feel utterly alone.

3

I left the endocrinologist's office and forced my way through the thick heat of the May afternoon and into the solitude of my car. The doctor had given me a prescription for an oral hypoglycemic, a pill that was supposed to lower my blood sugar level. He had also written down on a prescription pad the brand name of the type of glucose monitor I needed to buy and the type of test strips that were compatible with the monitor. I also had the pamphlets that he had given me.

Glancing at a folded strip of paper lying on the passenger seat of my sweltering car, I remembered that I had another prescription, written earlier that day by my gynecologist, for a medicine to treat my recurring yeast infection. Until I saw that prescription, I had forgotten all about the ailment which had started the whole sequence of events. Had that appointment really only been this morning? It seemed so long ago.

Armed with the prescriptions and informational brochures, I was naively confident, even though I was also overheated, overtired, and pretty much overwhelmed. All I needed to do was drive to the drugstore, get my prescriptions filled, and buy a glucose monitor. Then I could go home. I would figure out the monitor, read the brochures, and start to get a handle on this thing after I got home. I was sure I could have it all figured out before nightfall.

As it turned out, though, it was nearly nightfall before I had even secured all of my supplies. The prescriptions were easy enough, but the glucose monitor turned out to be a greater challenge. In a locked glass cabinet at the pharmacy counter of my local drugstore, I identified the brand the endocrinologist had recommended. I waited my turn in line and finally told a cashier that I needed one of the glucose monitors from that locked cabinet. "Sure, I can get that for you," he said. "Can I see your prescription?"

"I need a prescription? I don't have a prescription. My doctor just wrote the name for me on this piece of paper, but it's not a prescription." A slight twinge of panic struck me as the line behind me grew.

"You can buy one without a prescription, but it's not going to be covered by insurance. You can file for it later and see if your insurance company pays." The clerk was trying to be helpful, and I was trying to stay focused, despite my rising anxiety.

"Well, let me see, how much is it?" I asked as the clerk and I bent down together to try to read the price tag on the edge of the shelf beneath the display model.

"It looks like this one is $64.99. And you'll need the test strips," he added.

"Test strips? It doesn't come with those?"

"It comes with five or ten," he answered. "Are you going to need more than that?"

"I don't know. I can always come back for those, right?"

"Oh, yes. We have them right here. Let's see.... We have vials of fifty test strips for $34.99."

"And do I need a prescription for those?"

"You do if you want your insurance to cover them."

I couldn't do the exact math easily in my head, but it sounded like roughly the amount I had in my checking account at the time. I was supposed to test my glucose levels four times day. At that rate, a vial of fifty strips would last me about a week and a half. I was about to learn one of the first lessons of having a chronic health condition: It's expensive to be sick.

I told the clerk that I'd just buy the monitor, with however many test strips were included. I could buy additional test strips later if I needed them. At that early point, I couldn't comprehend that I would always need test strips. Ten test strips, if that was how many were included with the monitor, would last me about two days. I didn't understand then that I'd need more the day after that, and more the day after that, and more the day after that, and so on, for the rest of my life.

"Let me go in back and get you this monitor. The one on the shelf here is just an empty box for the display," the clerk told me.

I stepped aside and let the person behind me take my place at the counter. I found myself in front of a display rack of medical identification bracelets. The bracelets featured industrial-strength chains attached to metal ovals that were decorated with a red health insignia on the front side. The back of each one bore the name of a different medical condition in all capital letters: ALLERGIES, ANGINA, ASTHMA, and so on, alphabetically down the line. There, right after several cardiac listings, was the name of my new disease: DIABETES. I had just removed the DIABETES bracelet from its rack and was pondering what message this word on a bracelet conveyed, when the clerk returned. I put the bracelet back.

"We don't have that monitor in stock," he told me. "But I called our other store, and they have one. They're holding it for you." I thus was instructed in lesson number two of having a chronic health condition: There are a lot of logistical complications to being sick. You need what you need when you need it, regardless of whether it's covered by insurance and regardless of whether it's in stock. You have to find what you need, and you have to be able to pay for it.

Fortunately, the question-and-answer session about the glucose monitor lasted long enough that the pharmacist had the time to fill my two prescriptions. The clerk rang the prescriptions up and told me the total.

"Can I add one thing?" I asked. I reached over, grabbed the DIABETES bracelet, and added it to my purchase.

As I finally walked into my apartment that evening, my telephone was ringing. As much as I wanted to talk to Paul, if that's who was calling, I didn't have the energy to rush over and answer it. I plopped down on the couch, let the phone ring, and tried to decide what to do first. Read the pamphlets? Take my new diabetes pill? Treat the yeast infection? Figure out my monitor? Crawl under the bed and never come out?

The phone, which had stopped ringing, started ringing again just a moment later, and I thought I'd better answer it.

"Hello?" I said, making a conscious effort to sound normal, whatever "normal" now was for me.

I heard my mother's voice. "Well, hello there. I just called and didn't leave you a message. You know I don't like talking into your answering machine. I'm just not comfortable leaving messages on those machines. I want to leave a message with a person, not a machine. But you don't have any roommates, so there's nobody to leave a message with. And you always tell me I should leave a message if you don't answer, so I was calling back to leave you a message, but now you answer the phone. Were you screening your calls? You told me once that you screen your calls sometimes."

I took a deep breath. "Hi, Mom. No, I wasn't screening my calls. I just walked in the door, literally."

"This is late for you to get home from work, isn't it?" She was right, but it was utterly baffling to me how she knew that this was late for me to get home from work. "Did you have something to do?"

"No, I was barely at work today. I've been running around to doctor appointments all day. And then I had to go to a couple of drug stores to pick up prescriptions and get some other stuff. So I'm just getting home from all of that."

"Doctor appointments? Is everything okay?"

"Not really. No, I don't think everything is okay," I said. Being accustomed to all sorts of tales of medical woe by virtue of her career in nursing, my mother often shares clinical horror stories as an almost reflexive response when she hears news about anyone's health. I knew that when I shared my news, I could be potentially opening the floodgates. Taking another deep breath, I said, "I have diabetes."

"Diabetes? Well, what do the doctors say about it? Is it Type 1 or Type 2? Are they going to start you on insulin?"

"The doctor thinks I'm Type 2," I said. "He doesn't think I'm going to need insulin. He prescribed a pill that I'm starting on tonight. That should lower my glucose levels. He told me to get a glucose monitor, which I did, and I'm also supposed to check my glucose levels four times a day. I go back to see him the first of next week."

"Well, thank goodness they don't think it's Type 1." And then she barreled straight down the clinical horror story route. She didn't do it because she was unsympathetic or uncaring. She did it because she wanted to say that a lot of bad things have happened to other people, but they won't happen to me. The problem was that she always forgot to say the part about them not happening to me.

"I don't know if you remember that nurse who worked with me on West 2 when you were little? You might remember her—she was kind of plump, pretty, always wore her hair in a braid down her back? She had the thickest, reddest hair. Anyway, she was Type 1. And she just knew that it was going to be too risky for her ever to have kids, so she made the decision to go ahead and have a hysterectomy when she was about your age. No, she would've been a little younger than you, but she just thought she would go ahead and have her uterus taken out, so there was no chance of her ever even getting pregnant. But I can't imagine they would suggest anything like that for you. That was twenty-five years ago."

No, they won't suggest that for me. But thanks for mentioning it. Thanks for planting that particular seed.

"Now there's this other gal," she continued, "maybe I've told you about her. I met her through the health ministry at the church. She's Type 1, and her diabetes got so bad that she went blind. She lives alone, and I think she gets along pretty well, but she can't fill her insulin syringes herself, and she needs help getting her groceries. So I go over once a week and fill her syringes for the week and take her to the grocery store. She lives over near the...."

My mother continued to talk, but I could no longer process what I was hearing. I waited for her to finish up.

"Amy, are you still there? You haven't said anything."

"Yes, I'm here." How could I end this? I thought fast and said, "My other line was just beeping. It's probably Paul. He's out of town, and he must be wondering where I've been. Let me grab the other line, and I'll call you back in a few days when I know more." I hung up the phone, silencing her cautionary tales of hysterectomies and blindness.

I slumped down into the couch again, utterly exhausted and not knowing what to do next. Then I remembered that I needed to check my messages. That's what I would do next. One thing at a time. *Please, please, please,* I thought to myself, *let there be one from Paul.* And indeed, providing me with the only objective evidence I had seen all day that life was not cruel, I had one message, and it was from Paul. He had tried to reach me several times at my office, and he was wondering where I had been all day. He said he'd call me back, probably around 10. It was about 8:45 then, so 10:00 would be perfect. That would give me time to get a handle on things and be a little more informed when I talked to him. I wanted to understand diabetes better when he asked me about it. Surely an hour would be enough time for me to figure that out.

I went to the kitchen, took one of my new diabetes pills, and swallowed it down with a full glass of water. Feeling satisfied that I had checked one item off my new to-do list, I settled myself on the couch and resolved to figured out my new glucose meter. I opened the box and was surprised to find more than a few different components inside: there was the meter itself, which looked vaguely similar to the one I had seen in my gynecologist's office; another long, tubular device, the purpose of which was not immediately apparent to me; a bottle of something labeled "Control Solution"; a small plastic bag containing several pin-sized, plastic-encased items; a vial containing the ten test strips that had been the subject of my conversation with the clerk at the drug store; and a thick instruction manual. There was nothing intuitive about any of these devices or the relationship of any one thing in the box to any of the others. With a heavy sigh, I withdrew the instruction manual, opened it up, and perused the table of contents.

"Getting Started." That was what I needed: to get started. Step 1—Check the Contents of Your Package. This section listed, without the benefit of a diagram, the same number of items I had found inside the package. At least the numbers matched up—that was a good sign. Using a process of elimination, I was able to determine what each item was. The long, tubular item that I had not recognized turned out to be the lancing device—in other words, the finger sticker. The small, pin-sized items were the lancets—the sharp instruments that are inserted into the lancing device, cocked back, and then released to pierce the skin and draw blood. The lancing device had a depth-selection gauge as well, ranging in scale from 1, for the user whose fingertips do not require a deep stick to draw blood, to 5, for the user whose skin has thickened from enduring tens of thousands of needle-sticks.

More than any of the other items in the box, the lancing device and the lancets were hard to contemplate. The finger sticks were going to hurt. That was clear to me. Not only were they going to hurt, they were going to be self-inflicted. I was going to have to load the lancing device, hold it against my skin, and pull the trigger. No matter how little I wanted to do it, no matter how much it hurt, I was going to have to do it. My throat closed slightly at the thought. Time to move on to the next step.

Having organized the contents of the package and loaded the lancing device with a sharp new lancet, I turned to Step 2—Coding Your Meter. Here the manual explained that the meter had to be coded to match a number on the vial of test strips that would be used with the meter. There was also a highlighted cautionary note: Failure to code the meter correctly could result in inaccurate test results. I examined the label on the vial of test strips and found that it contained many numbers—a lot number, a manufacturing date, an expiration date, a number indicating the quantity of test strips in the vial, a range of numbers indicated as the control solution range and, also clearly marked as such, a code number. So there it was, the code number.

I went on to the next instruction. "Turn on the meter and insert a test strip." That wasn't as easy as it sounded, because nothing on the meter was marked as the "on/off" switch. There was a button marked "M," a button marked "C," a "+" button, and a "-" button. None of these buttons seemed to designate on or off. I again reviewed the table of contents, and was referred to a diagram that identified the function of each of the keys on the meter. Still, nothing. The front inside cover of the manual listed a customer-service line available 24 hours a day to respond to questions about the meter. Could it be that I would have to call this number just to figure out how to turn my meter on?

Just as I was considering calling customer service, my telephone rang. I was so lost in the world of the glucose meter that for a moment, I thought it must be the customer-service department calling me to see if I had any questions. On my way to pick up the ringing phone, I glanced at the clock and realized it was nearly 10 p.m. Over an hour had passed since I had gotten home. That must be Paul calling, and I was no closer to having figured out my new situation than I was when I had gotten home. In fact, I felt farther away and more confused than ever.

"Hello?"

"Amy? Where have you been? I called the office, and they said you'd been out at the doctor's all day. What's going on?"

It was Paul. Thank God, it was Paul. I burst into tears. It's hard to imagine that there was ever a time when Paul had not heard me sob. Having now been married to me for over a decade and a half, and having weathered children, pets, jobs, homes, and countless other joys and sorrows, Paul now is not particularly disturbed by my tears when they come. Until that day in 1996, though, there had been nothing in my life with Paul that had brought me to choking tears. But there I found myself, alone in my apartment, unable to answer his question, sobbing nearly convulsively.

"Amy, what's going on? Are you okay?" A little stern now.

"I have diabetes," I blurted out between sobs.

"You have what?" he asked, confused.

"Diabetes," I nearly screamed. "I have diabetes."

There was a pause while he collected his thoughts and I continued to cry. "What does that mean?" he asked gently.

"I don't know what it means. I don't know. Oh, my God, I don't know what any of this means." I was screaming now. Screaming and crying.

"Do you want me to come home?" he asked.

I didn't know what to say. I wanted a lot of things. I wanted to figure out my meter. I wanted the pill that I had taken to work. I wanted it to be yesterday, last week, last month, any day before today. I wanted Paul to come home, but I didn't tell him so.

"I'm coming home," he said, the sternness gone from his voice. "I'll take the first shuttle back in the morning. Now tell me what you know."

I told Paul what I knew about my condition, which at that point was not very much. I had so many more questions than answers. The answers could take time, he assured me, and I was not going to figure them all out that night. All I really needed to do that night was understand how to work the glucose meter so I could check my glucose level before I went to bed. If I could just do that, I could go to sleep and try to answer some of my other questions tomorrow.

After I calmed down a little, Paul got more comfortable. He wanted my assurance that I wasn't going to do anything other than figure out my glucose meter and then go to bed. I wasn't going to worry. I wasn't going to prognosticate. I wasn't going to assume the worst. I was just going to figure out how to prick my finger, get my glucose level, and then go to bed. I did feel calmer, and I did believe that I could get through the next twelve hours until he got back to town. We said good night, and I hung up the phone. With new resolve, I turned back to my glucose meter.

After thumbing through a few other sections of the instruction manual, I discovered that the meter did not actually have an on/off switch. The meter turned on whenever a test strip was inserted, and it turned off when the test strip was removed. The "M" and "C" buttons had to do with the meter's memory and recordkeeping functions, and the "+" and "-" keys were for programming the code number for the test strips.

Following the instructions, I inserted a test strip and pressed the "+" button until the number displayed on the screen of the glucose monitor matched the code number on the container of test strips. Once the meter was coded, a teardrop-shaped image representing a drop of blood began to blink on the screen, indicating that the meter was ready to receive a drop of blood. Gritting my teeth, I cocked the lancet device, placed it against my fingertip, and pulled the trigger. I felt a sting, but when I removed the device from my finger there was no blood. My fingertip was slightly inflamed from where it had been stuck, but there was no discernible blood.

I cranked up the lancet depth level to 2 and tried again on another fingertip. A nearly imperceptible drop of blood appeared on this fingertip. I squeezed my fingertip, as instructed by the manual, to try to get a bigger drop of blood to form. The squeezing caused the drop to get a little bigger. I rubbed the drop against the test strip that was inserted into the meter. The meter beeped when the blood came in contact with the test strip, and the display on the screen switched from a drop of blood to an hourglass. I waited for the result to be displayed on the screen, which the manual told me would take approximately twenty seconds. Just a few seconds later, the meter beeped again, and the screen displayed "Er5."

What is "Er5?" Even as a novice, I knew this wasn't a glucose level. I discerned that it must be an error message of some sort, and I flipped distractedly through the instruction manual to try to find an explanation. It wasn't long before I gave up on flipping through the manual and decided to call the customer-service line. There were a lot of things I didn't understand about my new glucose meter, so I might as well just get the folks who knew what they were doing to walk me through it all on the phone.

I called the toll-free number and was connected with a member of the customer-service staff. I explained that I was new to the glucose-testing world, and I told him about the "Er5" display on the screen of my glucose meter.

"That's an error message," he told me "It means you didn't get enough blood on the test strip."

"Not enough blood?" I asked, confused. "How much do you need?"

"You really need a good hanging drop. Look at the illustration on page 12 of your manual."

I turned to page 12. There was an illustration under the heading "Right" showing a fingertip with a round, full, tear-shaped drop of blood dangling from it, barely able to hang on. Lower down the page was an illustration under the heading "Wrong" that showed a smear of blood on a fingertip, just a stain really, ready to be rubbed against the test strip. The blood depicted in the "Wrong" illustration was much closer to what I had dabbed onto the test strip than the heavy drop depicted in the "Right" illustration.

"Well, now that I see these drawings, I see what I did wrong," I said to the service rep. "So what do I do now?"

"All you need to do is take out the old test strip, put in a new one, and try again. You need to get a better drop of blood."

"Right," I said slowly, pondering that concept. A better drop of blood. The phrase seemed nonsensical to me. What had happened during this day that found me now at home alone, feeling very nervous, talking on the phone to a stranger about the quality of a drop of my blood? I felt outside myself. Or not at all myself. I was beginning to come apart. I thought about the test strip that I had just been told to discard. It was one of ten. I had nine left. After this test I would have eight. What a waste. What if I went through the next eight test strips so carelessly?

"Can you stay on the phone while I try again?" I asked. It was nice having someone on the phone. It was nice not to be alone. "I'm not really sure what I'm doing."

"Oh sure, that's not a problem. Just take your time," he answered. "And this time, before you start, let your hand hang down by your side for a few seconds, and then squeeze your fingertip until it's really red. Then lance it. That should get you a good drop."

I did as instructed. When my fingertip was red, I pulled back the trigger on the lancing device, placed it against my finger tip, and pulled the trigger. Bingo. I had a nice red dangling drop of blood right way. "Oh," I exclaimed into the phone. "I think this one looks good. What do I do now?"

"Now lightly touch the blood onto the test strip. Don't touch the strip with your finger, though—you just want the blood. Don't smear the blood on the test strip. If you touch it lightly, the whole drop should fall away and stay on the test strip."

Again I did as instructed. Just as the service rep had predicted, the full drop of blood detached from my fingertip and filled the testing area on the strip. I could immediately see the difference between this drop of blood and the first one I had tried. There, finally, I had learned something: You need a good drop of blood for the glucose tests.

"This looks good," I said to the customer-service guy. "I've got the hourglass now," I remarked, referring to the display on the screen.

"Okay. Now it should just take about twenty seconds for your glucose level to show."

I waited while the hour glass blinked. Finally the glucose meter beeped, and then displayed a number: 377. A cautionary note flashed at the bottom of the display screen: "Test for ketones!" I didn't know what to do or say. This certainly was not the result I was hoping for, especially after having taken my new pill. I could not expect the pill to have started working in just a few hours, but why was my glucose level higher than it had been earlier in the day, when it was already at a level that several doctors found alarming?

The service rep brought me back to the conversation. "Did I hear your meter beep? Did you get your result?"

"I did get my result. Yes, I did."

"What was it?"

"Three hundred seventy-seven," I answered

"Did you say 377?" He stopped being my friendly customer-service representative and turned into an automaton. His next comments sounded as if he were reading from a script. "That is a dangerously high glucose level. You need to follow the high blood sugar protocol given to you by your doctor."

"I don't have a protocol," I said. "I don't know what I'm supposed to do. I just found out today that I have diabetes. I don't know anything about any of this." I couldn't have sounded, or felt, more desperate.

"You need to contact your personal physician. You should seek medical assistance immediately. I cannot give you medical advice."

Our relationship had changed. He was not comfortable talking to me any longer. I had hit the wall with him. There was no point in asking him for further advice. "Thanks very much for your help," I said, and I laid down the phone.

I felt mildly panicked, not knowing what to do about this 377, not understanding whether I was in any immediate danger. Then I remembered my friend Spratley. She was one of my oldest and dearest friends, and she happened to live just a short drive away. Spratley also happened to work for a communications and advertising firm, and I remembered her mentioning recently that she had put together an informational video on diabetes for a client. Why had I not thought

SHOT

of her earlier? She'd know what I should do. I knew it was a little late, but I dialed her number anyway.

"Sprat?"

"Hey, what's going on?" she answered. It was clear by the sound of her voice that I had woken her. It was, after all, past eleven at night.

"Oh, Spratley, I'm freaking out. I am *really* freaking out," I began.

"Why? What happened?" By the sound of her voice, I could tell she was getting out of bed, springing to action, ready to right whatever had wronged me. Everyone should have a friend like Spratley.

"I don't know what happened... I mean, I have diabetes. I found out today that I have diabetes."

"I'll be right there. Give me ten minutes. Ten minutes, okay?" Oh, God bless her. Surely I could hang on for ten more minutes. "Oh, I wish I were still within pajama-walking distance. I'll be right there." And she hung up.

She had tried to lighten the mood with her pajama-walking comment. Several years after college, we had by chance ended up living in the same city, in apartments less than a block apart. Each of us had on occasion, late at night after a spat with a boyfriend or early in the morning in desperate need of a cup of coffee, walked to the other's apartment in pajamas.

So with Spratley now driving-distance away, I had a few minutes to fill before she would arrive. I decided to delve into one of my pamphlets, hoping again to garner some new understanding of my condition and hoping to be more collected when Spratley arrived.

I assembled my pamphlets in a semicircle around me on the couch. Which to read first? How about "Diabetes and You?" That seemed to sum up the present company, so I figured that was as good a place as any to start.

The pamphlet was written in an easily understandable prose but should have borne a warning label, so frightening were its contents. After a brief introductory note to remind me that I had been diagnosed with the disease, the pamphlet proceeded to list the possible complications of uncontrolled diabetes: ketoacidosis, heart disease, blindness, nerve damage, and kidney damage. Incongruously, the complications were listed beneath a photograph of an apparently healthy 20-something-year-old woman perched atop the shoulders of an equally hale young man, spiking a volleyball over a net in a swimming pool game. It was not clear what role diabetes played in their lives, but it was clear that it was not going to interfere with their game of volleyball.

The next page featured a speedometer-style graph that was divided into green, yellow and red areas based on glucose levels. Green, as in "full speed ahead, take life by the horns," was for glucose levels from 90 to 115. Yellow, as in "caution, pay attention to your glucose levels," was for glucose levels from 115 to 200. Red, as in "alert, danger zone," was for glucose levels above 200. I was deep into the red zone.

The brochure also had a note on ketoacidosis, one of the complications of diabetes. I realized upon seeing the word in print that this was the term that had been batted around about me earlier in the day at my general practitioner's office. Ketoacidosis, the brochure explained, is diabetic coma. Ketoacidosis develops when the body does not have enough insulin and begins to break down fats. This produces a waste product called ketones. *This must be why I've been losing weight*, I thought to myself. According to the brochure, when ketones build up in the blood, the body tries to rid itself of the ketones through urine. *This must be why I've been peeing so often.* When there are high levels of ketones in the urine, the body cannot release them all, and they build up to dangerous levels in the bloodstream.

At that point in the brochure, this cautionary note to the reader might have been in order: "Read no further if you are home alone, newly diagnosed, and prone to hypochondriacal flights of fancy." The brochure went on to explain that ketoacidosis is a life-threatening condition that requires immediate medical attention. There followed a bullet-point list of symptoms of ketoacidosis that included:

- shortness of breath (upon reading this, I found myself gulping for air, unable to take a deep breath)
- fruity-smelling breath (I blew, with what I believed was the scarce breath remaining in me, into the cupped palm of my hand and detected the distinct aroma of strawberries)
- nausea and vomiting (my stomach churned and cramped)
- a very dry mouth (my tongue swelled to three times its normal size and stuck to the sandpaper roof of my mouth)

The lines of text in the brochure became wavy. Squinting through what I now believed were diabetes-damaged eyes, I could not make sense of any it. The letters swam and lifted off the page. I put down the brochure, picked up the remote control, and tried to turn on the television to distract myself. I aimed the remote and looked across the room at the television. Its formerly well-defined metal edges had become soft and curvy, as fluid as the lines of text in the brochure I had been reading. The screen bubbled out.

I dropped the remote and picked up the phone. I needed to get help. I believed that I was succumbing to a diabetic coma. I couldn't wait any longer for Spratley to arrive. With an index finger that seemed to extend far from my hand and to curve adroitly, I chased down and captured the digits "9," "1," and "1" as they flew off the number pad and tried to get away.

I slumped back into the couch and waited for the ambulance to arrive. In the few minutes that passed between when I called Spratley and when she actually arrived, I forgot that I had even called her. I was startled when there was a knock at my door and Spratley let herself in. The scene that greeted her surprised her. We had not seen each other in a few weeks, and I had lost a lot of weight. I was skinny—not a good-looking, healthy kind of skinny, but a bony kind of skinny. My apartment was in shambles, too, and that was unusual for me. Spratley found me there on my couch, wide-eyed and scared, surrounded by brochures, a bottle of pills, a prescription bag, scattered, small-type warning inserts, a glucose meter with its many accoutrements, and clutching the phone.

"I called 911," I said by way of greeting.

"Okay, good. How do you feel?" she asked.

"I feel dizzy. I just feel very out of it," I responded, "but I do feel a little better than I did when I called the emergency number." Indeed, just knowing that there were trained medical professionals on the way had given me some reassurance.

"You're dizzy. You need orange juice. Do you have any orange juice?" Spratley asked.

"I don't know if I do. Why do I need orange juice?"

"It was in that diabetes video that I made at work—if you feel dizzy or shaky, that means your blood sugar is too low and you need orange juice to bring it back up," she explained without breaking stride as she moved toward my kitchen and zeroed in on the refrigerator.

"But my blood sugar isn't too low. It's too high. I don't think I'm supposed to have anything with sugar in it right now."

Spratley stopped searching for the orange juice, peered over the refrigerator door, and asked, "Too high? What are you supposed to do if it is too high? Did the doctor give you insulin?"

"No, I don't have to take insulin. I took a pill..." Before I could launch into another explanation of how I didn't understand what was happening to me, the paramedics arrived at my apartment. They ushered me into the ambulance and drove me to the local hospital. Spratley followed in her car.

The paramedics quizzed me on the way to the hospital, and I answered them as if I was living inside a dream:

"How long have you had diabetes?"

About twelve hours, to my knowledge.

"Do you know what your glucose level is?"

Three hundred seventy-seven.

"Did your doctor give you any instructions about how to treat high blood sugar?"

He prescribed a pill.

"Do you know whether you have ketones in your urine?"

Earlier in the day I did, and my glucose level has gone higher since then.

"What have you had to eat or drink in the past few hours?"

I don't remember eating or drinking anything all day.

"How do you feel now?"

Here, in this emergency vehicle, surrounded by licensed medical practitioners, I feel fine. I'm no longer dizzy. I can breathe. My mouth isn't so dry. I feel like I might pull through.

Arriving at the emergency room, I learned another important fact about having diabetes: It puts you high up on the triage list. I was immediately taken back to a bed in a holding area of the emergency ward and given an IV with fluids in it. It had not occurred to me until the paramedics had asked that I probably had not had anything to eat or drink that whole day. That was unusual for me. Underweight though I was, I routinely ate at least three squares a day and drank a lot of water.

The emergency room staff also checked my glucose level regularly. It hovered in the 370s. They let Spratley come back and stay with me. After a few hours, at about two in the morning, one of the nurses came back and told me they were going to unhook me and send me home. I was stunned. *They were sending me home? How could I go home? I didn't know how to take care of myself. I didn't know how to get my glucose level out of the 370s.*

While I was being transported to the emergency room in the ambulance and while I was lying on my emergency room bed staring at the ceiling in my holding bay, snippets of conversations that I had heard but never contemplated at various times throughout my life flitted in and out of my head.

They found out she had diabetes. She was in the hospital for a few days until they got it regulated.... They had him in the hospital until they got his diabetes under control.

I had convinced myself that they were going to keep me there until I understood how to manage my diabetes. And I was fine with that. Let me stay in the hospital for weeks, if that was what it would take. Just do not send me home to try to figure it out alone. But sending me home was exactly what they were doing.

"Yup, you're good to go. Call your doctor in the morning and tell him about your glucose levels tonight, but we're done with you," the attendant told me cheerfully.

Spratley saw the panic on my face. "I'll take you home to my house. You can't say no. You're staying with me tonight."

4

What sent me to the hospital that night had nothing to do with diabetes. I learned in the emergency room that there was nothing wrong with me. Well, there was nothing *new* wrong with me, anyway. I still had the diagnosis itself to grapple with, but there was nothing other than the diabetes. There was no blurry vision. There were no heart palpitations. There was really no confusion in my mind. Other than my soaring blood glucose level, there was nothing physically wrong with me. That's why they had sent me home.

I insisted that my symptoms must have been a side effect of the pill that I had taken only minutes before the onset. "That's unlikely," the emergency room doctor said. "Those aren't typical side effects. It might be a case of the nerves. That would be completely understandable."

Nerves? He was telling me this was nerves? That was a little insulting. I had just learned in the course of one day that I might go blind, my kidneys might fail, and I might never be able to have a baby. And this guy was telling me that I had a case of the nerves? The outrage of it all was enough to stun me back to some level of stability.

None of the doctors whom I would see over the next few weeks would confirm what I knew to be the case: That I had broken into a cold sweat, that my vision had been swimming, and that my heart had been racing because I was about to drop dead on the floor. They all said the same thing. I was likely suffering from anxiety, and I had probably suffered a panic attack. And thus I was introduced to another new reality that I could have lived comfortably without: Failings of the mind are every bit as powerful as failings of the body and sometimes harder to control.

People who have diabetes suffer from anxiety and depression at a rate that can be twice as high as the population at large. Symptoms of those conditions can confound a person with diabetes, because so many mimic the symptoms or complications of diabetes. Breaking into a sudden sweat? It could be low blood sugar, or it could be your mind. Too tired to drag yourself out of bed? It could be high blood sugar, or it could be your mind. Tightness in your chest? It could be heart disease, or it could be your mind. Tingling in your feet? It could be neuropathy, or it could be your mind.

Those of us who have diabetes do not have a corner on the market for depression and anxiety. Chronic disease sufferers of all sorts find their physical ailments compounded by the psychic weight of it all. The prevalence of anxiety and depression in association with chronic medical illness is a well-documented phenomenon. So maybe people who have diabetes haven't cornered the market, but we do have a special top-shelf area for those who know what a glucose level is, for those who have had a glucose level so low they could not tell you their home address, and for those who have had a glucose level so high they have fallen into a coma.

Why shouldn't we feel overwhelmed and anxious? Type 1 diabetes is a relentless disease that does not let you rest. It doesn't let you forget about it, even for an afternoon. Type 2 diabetes is a scourge all its own, letting you ignore it for a while if you choose and then catching up with you later, as you always knew it would. Gestational diabetes has its own class of fear: the knowledge that the life of your baby depends every day on your glucose level. It is exhausting not to get a break. It's hard to worry about complications, and it's torture to fret about the life developing inside of you.

All these years later I have found that it's not always easy, nor is there always time, to talk about mental health issues with my diabetes doctor. There is enough to cover at my appointments already—pages and pages of glucose levels to wade through, lab results to discuss, vision screenings to be done, blood to be drawn, urine samples to be given. On occasions where I have raised it with my doctor—"Uh, doctor, I've been feeling a little nervous lately... I can't seem to stop worrying about a low..."—I have sometimes gotten a bit of a brush-off response: "That's understandable. Anyone in your shoes is going to worry about that a little." Once, rather than the brush-off, I actually got a referral to a therapist. *Right*, I thought upon receiving the referral. *I will simply add a therapist to the team of people trying to keep me healthy.*

People who have diabetes are advised to have a whole host of physicians and other specialists at the ready: an endocrinologist, a general practitioner, an ophthalmologist, a podiatrist, a dentist, a registered dietician, perhaps a cardiologist or a nephrologist as well. The thought of adding a new member to my growing cadre of health care professionals just increased the stress I was already feeling. How could I add one more appointment to my schedule? How could I miss another afternoon of work? How could I file one more out-of-network insurance claim? And those thoughts heaped on more stress. But I did go to see the therapist. I needed to talk to someone about something other than my glucose levels.

She kept me waiting longer than I would have liked, emerging from her office and inviting me in nearly thirty minutes after my appointed time. "Sorry I kept you waiting. Tell me a little about your-self. What brings you in today?"

I decided to start off with a joke. "Well, good thing I'm not here, because people who are late drive me crazy."

That comment drew a blank stare. She was not amused. I decided to try again. I told her the real reason I was there. I told her about my recent diabetes diagnosis. I told her about all of the scary things that could happen to me. I told her that I had always been a very independent person, never one to rely on others, and now I found myself afraid to sleep alone, afraid to drive alone, afraid of all kinds of day-to-day activities that wouldn't have made me blink in my old life.

She was quiet for a while as she considered what I had told her. She had heard only the tip of the iceberg, but even that gave her a lot to think about. "I can see why you're worried," she said at last.

That's the best you can do? I thought to myself. *You've got to give me something more than that.* But she had given me validation. At least she hadn't told me that I was nuts or that I really had nothing to be worried about.

"Have you ever taken medication for your anxiety?" she asked. I didn't like how she called it "my anxiety." It made it sound like a part of me, like something that had always been there. But it hadn't always been there. This was a new problem. This had come with the diabetes.

"No, I've never had this kind of problem before. This is new for me. But I don't want to take medication. There must be something I can do other than that." I had gone from being a person who took no medicine to being a person who took medication for diabetes and medication for an underactive thyroid (which was also discovered with my diabetes diagnosis). I didn't want to add a third type of medication, and I didn't want to hand over control of my emotions to a pill. There must be something I could still control on my own, without some extra medicine.

"Well, if you're sure you don't want to take anything, you can try some relaxation techniques."

"Okay, let's try that out. What do I do?"

"Close your eyes, and take a few deep breaths. Think of a time when you were very happy, when you were completely content and relaxed."

I couldn't think of anything that worked, because each thought that popped into my head was of the old me—the me who did not have diabetes. Happy thoughts about my old life weren't going to help. They weren't relevant, because my old life was gone. It made me sad to think of my formerly carefree self. That wasn't comforting in the least.

"I get the idea," I said, cutting short the exercise. "I can work on that. Is there anything else?"

"Well, are you allowed to drink wine? Maybe a glass of wine in the evening would help to relax you."

I smiled. That was the best advice I had gotten in ages.

Shortly after that appointment, I reached out to my mother, and, in a rare show of vulnerability, I told her how I was suffering. She suggested that I call one of our oldest and dearest family friends. This is a man whom I would trust with my life. A man whom, until my mother told me, I had never known had diabetes. What a glimmer of hope that was! I had spent many of the weekend nights of my teenage years babysitting for his children, I had gone to church with him for as long as I could remember. But I had never once imagined he had diabetes. That must be a positive: Surely it must mean you can have diabetes without constantly believing you're going to succumb to its complications.

"Amy," he said warmly when he heard my voice. "Hey, kid, your mom told me. I'm sorry to hear it. That's a tough thing. I know how tough it is."

"But Ed," my voice quaked, "I can't get control of myself. I can't stop worrying. I can't stop thinking something is going to happen to me."

Silence: Did he not know what to say?

"Did that ever happen to you?"

"No, not really."

Damn. Maybe somehow it hadn't been so tough for him? I pressed on, desperate for help.

"But how did you deal with it? Weren't you kind of scared? Weren't you confused?"

"Well," he began, "I certainly remember how hard it was at first. But I mostly remember feeling that I had so much to live for. Carolyn and I had just gotten married. I was in law school. I didn't concentrate on the worrying part. I just had to keep my life going, because I had so many good things to live for."

There was a thought: so much to live for—just as there was, legitimately, so much to be afraid of. But he had an important point: There was also so much *not* to be afraid of. At the time, my list of things to live for was objectively short. I had a boyfriend, a cat, an apartment, a car, and a job. When I broke it down, it was hard to latch on to any one of those things (save the boyfriend) as being enough to keep me going. But together didn't they add up to something? Cumulatively, didn't they point in the direction of someone who was starting to have a life? Maybe I could cope with diabetes because I did have so much to live for.

I didn't believe it would be easy, but it was something to think about at least. It was something I could shoot for. The next time the panic set in, the next time my heart beat like a rabbit's, the next time my field of vision narrowed, I would let it happen. I would let it wash over me, and I would tell myself that it would pass. And while it was passing, I would think of all I had to live for.

In the words of a dear friend who does not have diabetes but who has her own demons, I will just remember to breathe. And repeat. Breathe. Repeat.

5

I slept deeply in Spratley's guest room, if only for a few hours. It was nearly three in the morning by the time we got back to her house, and she had to get up for work at seven. She dropped me off at my apartment on her way to work. "Now you're going to be okay until Paul gets back, right?"

"I'll be fine. You're the best. I can never thank you enough for last night."

"Call me tonight," she instructed.

"I will. Thanks so much, Sprat. I don't know what might have happened if—"

"Stop thanking me. Bye."

And she was off. I trudged up the stairs to my apartment. I opened the door, which was unlocked. Apparently, I had neglected to lock it when the paramedics had taken me out the night before. I was greeted by the disarray that I had left behind: a prescription bottle, the instruction manual for my glucose meter, the cheery pamphlets, a box of alcohol swabs. It was all still there. My brief trip to the hospital hadn't made any of it go away.

I made my way through the debris and tried to start making some sense of it all. I put my pills away and then tucked my glucose meter into its carrying case. I stashed the extraneous equipment back in the box and made a mental note to figure it out later. I flipped through my pamphlets again and stacked them up in a neat little pile, ranked from least to greatest interest. Things looked better already. I looked at the clock. It was 8:30 in the morning. I still had half an hour until I could call the doctor's office, and an hour and a half until Paul arrived. Would a shower change anything important about me?

Since my diagnosis the day before, my world had been turned on its ear. Things that I had never thought twice about were now menacing: a bowl of cereal, a cup of coffee, a piece of toast. I didn't know the effect that any of these might have on my glucose level. I was afraid to eat or drink anything. But a shower? I probably could take a shower.

I emerged feeling refreshed. By the time I had dressed and brushed my teeth, it was after nine. Finally, I could call the doctor and tell him about my emergency room episode of last evening.

"Hello, yes, this is Amy Fitzgerald. I'm a new patient. I'd like to leave a message for the doctor, please." The receptionist put me on hold. She returned to the line a few minutes later and asked me if I could come in at eleven that morning to see the doctor.

"Yes, eleven is fine," I answered, encouraged that Paul would be back in time for the appointment He could help me figure this all out with the doctor. Now I was getting somewhere.

A short time later, Paul arrived at my apartment. I usually greeted him with at least a hug, quite often a kiss, and on occasion a true fantasy. So he was never sure what to expect. On this morning he was greeted by an unwelcome first—unvarnished fear. "Oh, thank God you're back," I said, burying my face in his chest. "I thought you'd never get here."

Paul came in, settled down with me on my couch, and listened patiently as I filled him in on the events of the past twelve hours. It was incomprehensible to me, after I broke it down, hour-by-hour, to realize that it had only been twelve hours since I had last talked to him. So much had happened in that time. And yet nothing had happened. I still didn't know what was wrong with me or how to fix it.

We went together to my doctor's appointment. It was the first time in many years that I had been to see a doctor in the company of someone who was taking some responsibility for my care. Rather than being offended at his paternalistic approach, as I would have been forty-eight hours earlier, I was comforted. *Thank goodness*, I thought to myself, *maybe the two of them can figure this out and just tell me what I need to do.*

I loved hearing myself referred to in the third person. When the doctor would say to Paul, for example, "Make sure she does this," or "Make sure she does that," they were talking about me as if I weren't there, and yet there I sat. It was marvelous. It was far too early for me to comprehend that no one was going to be able to fix this for me, that managing my diabetes would be up to me, and only me. And that always would be so.

I had lost another three pounds since meeting with the doctor just the day before. As the appointment wrapped up, the doctor rose and ushered us to the door. "Get her to eat. She's got to eat," he said as he shook Paul's hand and grasped his shoulder fondly.

"I will," Paul responded. He was happy to have an assignment from the doctor. If getting me to eat was his charge, then getting me to eat he would. We piled into Paul's car and headed toward his house.

"The doctor says you need to eat," he said as he drove, as if I had not heard the whole conversation. "Should we stop somewhere? Or can you think of something you want when we get back to my house?"

"I just want to sleep. I just want to put on my pajamas and sleep. I'll eat when I wake up. I promise. But right now I just want to sleep. I'm so tired."

He looked at me with concern. "Okay, baby. You can sleep. But when you wake up, you have to eat."

"I will, I swear," I assured him. After a pause I asked, "Will you stay with me while I sleep?" I was already afraid to sleep alone. I was starting to feel afraid of doing nearly anything alone. This was a foreign and unwelcome feeling for independent me.

"Of course I will." He looked at me again, concern in his eyes, and put his hand on my thigh. He could encircle almost all of it between his thumb and middle finger.

It was around noon when we got back to Paul's house. The heat had not broken. It was a soul-sapping exercise just to walk the thirty feet from his car to the front door. He had turned off the air conditioner before leaving town, and the house was stifling. As soon as we got inside, Paul switched on the window air-conditioning unit in the living room and dashed upstairs to turn on the one in his bedroom.

"It'll be cool in the bedroom in ten minutes," he announced as he floated down the stairs. Paul had then, and still has to this day, the ability to glide down a set of stairs without seeming to touch any one of them.

I was reassured by his news, not just because I wanted my sleeping chamber to be cool but because of what the air conditioner represented: a solution. There had been a problem—it was too hot in the house. Then there was a solution—turn on the air conditioner. I had a problem—I now have diabetes. There must be a solution—but what is it? The thought sapped more of my waning energy.

I managed to haul myself upstairs. I went into the bathroom to change into my pajamas. Paul thought it was funny that I was putting on pajamas in the middle of the day, but I wanted to wear them. I had bought them for our beach trip that now wouldn't happen. I changed and entered his small bedroom. It was nice and chilly. I pulled down the shades, climbed into bed, and buried myself under the sheets and blankets. Paul came in shortly afterward. He lay down on top of the covers, and wrapped his arms around the cocoon that contained me. I fell into the deepest sleep I would have for a long time.

I awoke a few hours later. Paul was there, keeping his patient vigil. I felt rested, groggy, and pleasantly disoriented. I looked at the clock on his bedside table. It read 4:15 PM. I noted the "PM" with confusion. I couldn't think why I had been sleeping so soundly at four o'clock in the afternoon. Then I remembered why I had been so tired. I remembered why I had slept for four hours in the middle of the day. "Oh God, honey," I moaned as the realization came back to me. I rolled over and buried my head under the pillows.

"I know, baby, I know." Then, not allowing me a moment more of self-pity, he said, "Come on, let's get up. Let's find something to eat." He pulled the blankets off and rousted me out of bed.

We drove into town. I didn't feel up to eating out, so we ordered carryout from an Italian restaurant that was one of our favorites. I wanted to be at Paul's house, and for the first meal that I would consume in more than twenty-four hours, I wanted comfort food—real Italian pizza made from scratch, with a thick, doughy crust and homemade tomato sauce.

When we were settled back at Paul's house, I ate one slice of pizza and washed it down with an ice cold glass of milk. It was simple fare, but it was extremely satisfying. The exercise of eating was good; it was normalizing. There—I had eaten dinner, and nothing bad had happened to me. *See,* I thought to myself, *you ate a yummy meal; your stomach is full; you're in the air-conditioned comfort of Paul's home; you're in love. This is all going to work out.*

The rest of the evening was quiet and comfortable. We watched television, cuddled together on the sofa, and even had a few laughs. Things were starting to feel almost normal. It had been a rough couple of days, but already I felt like I wasn't going to be derailed for long by my new condition. When the television program we were watching ended, we wandered upstairs to get ready for bed. Despite my long nap earlier that day, I was more than ready for another good sleep.

Paul got ready for bed first, and then it was my turn. I added my glucose meter to my assortment of overnight toiletries and headed into the bathroom to get ready for bed. "I'm going to check my glucose level before I come to bed," I said casually as I headed into the bathroom. I was trying to think of it as just another thing to do: wash face, brush teeth, check glucose. Surely I could add another item to my bedtime routine.

I had pricked my finger and successfully gotten a glucose reading several times since my initial call to the customer-service line the prior evening. All of my glucose readings had been in the high 200s or low 300s, still in the red zone, according to my diabetes pamphlet. So I was prepared for another high reading. The doctor had told me to expect this and not to be alarmed by it. I was on day two of the pill that the doctor had prescribed, which was supposed to lower my glucose level. If I had Type 2 diabetes, the doctor had told me, the pill would work. It might take a few days, but it would work.

I lanced my fingertip and produced a full drop of blood, which I touched lightly onto the test strip that I had inserted into my meter. It was a picture-perfect drop of blood and application to the test strip—no errors like the night before. I waited while the hourglass icon blinked on and off the screen. I looked away and challenged myself not to look at the screen while I waited for the result to come. I stared at the ceiling and counted in my head, one-thousand-one, one-thousand-two, one thousand-three, and finally—beep: my result was ready. I looked down at the screen and nearly collapsed at the number: 429.

Four hundred twenty-nine? I felt dizzy. The Earth lurched on its axis. I held on to the edge of the bathroom counter with both hands, palms against the cold tiles, blood trickling out of my fingertip. Four hundred twenty-nine. My diabetes pamphlets did not discuss any glucose level above 240. Anything above 240 was lumped in the red zone. How high above 240 could my glucose level go before I simply expired?

I paged frantically through the manual for my glucose meter, trying to find any information that might indicate that this glucose level of 429 was not going to spell the end of me. Not finding anything, I turned to the index. The only word that came to mind for me to search for in the index was "high"—as in, "my glucose level is very high." So I went to the Hs. I didn't find "high," but I did find "HI [message]" and a reference to page 49. I turned to page 49. There I found an explanation of the message that appears on a user's screen if the glucose level is above a certain level: HI. If "HI" appears on your screen, you are to drop everything and go immediately to your nearest emergency medical facility. On this particular meter, this message indicates that your glucose level is above 500.

So now I could infer that a glucose level could go at least as high as 500, and apparently a person at this level would still have wits enough to seek medical assistance. As disturbed as I was with my 429, I was also mildly relieved to learn that I had seventy-one points to go before I got a HI message. It was a tempered sense of relief, though, to feel that I might be okay only because I knew it was possible to be worse.

I packed up my glucose meter, finished getting ready for bed, and re-entered the air-conditioned comfort of Paul's bedroom. He could tell that something was wrong. When he had last seen me, just a few minutes before, as we exchanged places in the bathroom, it seemed like I was returning to my old self. I now appeared in his room, pretending to be calm, but with a face that was pale, eyes that were wide, and hands that were trembling. I explained to him what had happened. "What should I do? Should I call 911 again? Should I call the doctor?"

"I don't think you need to call 911. If the manual says 500 is the level when you should get help, then I don't think you need to call 911 right now." He thought for a moment and then said, "But you could call your doctor. Just have him paged. He can call you back." As the son of a physician, Paul understood that doctors' lives are all about being paged after hours.

I called the pager number that my new endocrinologist had given me, keyed Paul's telephone number into the pager system, and waited for the doctor to call back. When the doctor called, Paul answered and gave the phone to me. I told the doctor about my glucose level of 429.

"What did you eat for dinner tonight?" the doctor asked.

I told him about the slice of pizza and glass of milk.

"Pizza?" he exclaimed. "You didn't tell me you were going to eat pizza."

Why would I tell you that I was going to eat pizza? I wondered. *You never asked me what I was going to eat. You just told me to eat.* It's not as if I had eaten cake or candy or any of the other sugary foods that I knew were off-limits for people with diabetes. All I had done was eat a slice of pizza. Yet the doctor's tone of voice made it sound as though I'd gotten what I should have expected.

"Wha—what's wrong with pizza?" I stammered.

"What's wrong with pizza?" He chuckled aloud as he restated my question. I could hear him shaking his head. "Pizza—think about it. The crust is loaded with carbohydrates. The tomato sauce is loaded with sugar. Pizza always makes glucose levels soar in diabetics."

"Oh, sure, now that you've explained it that way, I guess it makes sense," I said. But it didn't make sense, although I said it did. None of it was making sense. "So do I need to be worried about my glucose level right now?"

"No, no, not at all. It's just the pizza," he answered.

"I'm sorry to have bothered you with this."

"It's no bother," he insisted. "It's a bit of a learning curve, but you'll get it."

I hung up the phone, stunned yet again. "What'd he say?" Paul asked.

I answered slowly, deliberately, as if in a trance "He said it was the pizza. I don't know if I can eat pizza anymore..." I felt a dense cloud of confusion descend upon me. It wasn't that I ate pizza all the time, and so I wondered what I'd eat now. It was just that pizza seemed like such a harmless thing to eat. If I couldn't eat that, what else could I not eat? If the bread in the crust and the tomato sauce were enough to send my blood sugar through the roof, what did that mean for the rest of my diet?

I consulted my stack of pamphlets, which I had brought with me to Paul's house, and learned the most common misconception about diabetes: It's not about sugar. It's about carbohydrates. All carbohydrates break down into glucose. If diabetes were just about simple sugars, I could live with that. It wouldn't be fun to forego dessert after a nice dinner, a soda on a hot day, or candy on Halloween, but I could do it. Diabetes, however, wasn't so simple. Diabetes wasn't just about skipping dessert.

Diabetes is about carbohydrates. And carbohydrates are not just in desserts. Carbohydrates are everywhere. At breakfast, carbohydrates are in cereal, in the splash of milk in your coffee, in toast, in grapefruit, in bagels, in orange juice. At a midmorning snack, carbohydrates are in crackers, in fruit, in granola bars, in yogurt, in trail mix. At lunch, carbohydrates are in bread, in buns, in wraps, in salad dressings, in chips, in croutons. At dinner, carbohydrates are in pasta, in rice, in taco shells, in potatoes, in vegetables, in sauces, in wine. Diabetes is not about avoiding sweets. Diabetes is about understanding how many grams of carbohydrate are in every bite of food that you eat, and in every ounce of liquid that you drink, and what that will do to your glucose level. This could take a very long time to figure out. This could take a lifetime.

Paul and I spent what should have been our getaway weekend quietly. Our only social outing was at the home of his brother and sister-in-law for dinner with them and another couple, and then going to see a movie afterwards. They knew about my recent diagnosis and were eager to help me get my mind off my troubles. Although it had been only two days, Paul was concerned about how I was coping, or not coping, and he was happy to get me out of the house and try to distract me.

We explained to the other couple at dinner that I wasn't quite myself. I had just been diagnosed with diabetes, and I was still figuring out what was and was not off-limits. They were sympathetic to my new condition. They exhibited the response that I have come to know well over the years: genuine concern, along with no real understanding of what any of it meant.

My sister-in-law was, as always, a consummate hostess, but from the array of food that was offered, I chose to eat only carrots. Carrots seemed the one safe bet at that point. As we talked about the events of my last forty-eight hours, everyone became very curious about my glucose meter. Before the age of the cell phone, the Blackberry, and the iPod, my glucose meter was indeed something of a technological marvel.

I was happy to show it off. I was happy to be in the role of instructor. I had been bombarded with new information, and I was exhausted from playing the part of the new initiate, so I was thrilled to take the advisory role and tell everyone what they needed to know about a glucose meter. It gave me confidence to know more about my new condition than everyone else did.

They all wanted to test their glucose levels. That sounded like a great idea to me. I had been enlightened about my glucose level; shouldn't they be as well? I explained to everyone what a normal glucose level was, and then I cautioned them all not to be alarmed if their glucose levels were elevated. After all, they had eaten appetizers and a full meal, they had drunk beer and wine, and they had all eaten dessert. I didn't want them to be as shocked as I had been when their high glucose levels were revealed. I was not out to ruin anyone's night.

After putting a new lancet in the lancing device, I inserted a new test strip into the meter, pricked the finger of the first volunteer, and guided his finger to the test strip. The application was successful; the hour glass ticked; the familiar beep sounded. We all looked at the screen: 94. The grouped cheered. "Ninety-four. Hey, buddy, you're normal; you don't have diabetes." The group's elation was my consternation. *Ninety-four? After all that food? He must have an exceptionally active pancreas*, I thought. Paul was watching me nervously.

We went through the same exercise with the man's wife. Her finger prick yielded an 87. Again the group cheered at her normal glucose level. *Who was this couple with such freakishly normal glucose control?* I wondered. *Wasn't anyone going to have a high glucose level after all of the food and wine they'd just consumed?*

Our hosts pricked their fingers next in turn and got readings of 92 and 96. The volunteers congratulated each other on their fine glucose levels, compared the state of their punctured fingertips, and then realized that Paul had not yet tested his glucose level. "Okay, Ryan, it's your turn," they said, turning to Paul.

Paul looked at me and saw that my mood had shifted. This had been a bad idea. This little game had shown me that most people can eat and drink as they wish without a noticeable effect on their glucose levels. This had shown me that there was a huge and, to my mind, frightening difference between these people and me.

"I'm going to pass," Paul said. "Call me a wimp, but I hate blood." He was trying hard to change the subject, to steer everyone away from this newfound curiosity about glucose levels. "We should get going to the movies anyway. Parking is going to be tough." Paul was trying to get us out of the house before anyone noticed that I was about to lose it. The lump in my throat was nearly choking me. The tears pooling in my eyes wouldn't stay contained for long.

"If you're worried about parking, let's all drive together," one of our party offered.

"No, we'll drive separately," I blurted out. "I'm really tired. I might not make it through the movie." No one questioned me.

As soon as we closed the door and were in the privacy of Paul's car, I fell apart. He knew it was coming. "Oh my God, there's something really wrong with me. There's something really wrong..." I choked out the words through my sobs. "How did they get a 94? An 87? Oh my God, I must be sick—I must be really sick."

6

The rest of the holiday weekend passed between finger pricks. I had used up my first ten glucose test strips by the third day after my diagnosis, and I had gone back to the drugstore and shelled out $34.99 for another fifty. There were still a few kinks to work out, but I was getting much better at the art of glucose testing. The lowest reading I got all weekend was in the mid-200s. It did not appear that the pill I was taking was working.

Finally, after three long days, none of which was spent at the beach, Memorial Day weekend was over. I was relieved when Tuesday morning rolled around, as this was the day that I was to return to the endocrinologist and report on my glucose levels. As the doctor looked through the booklet in which I had logged my readings for the past few days, he seemed mildly concerned. "Hmmm," he mused, shaking his head ever so slightly as he flipped through the pages of my log. "I would've expected to see lower readings than this. Looks like this pill might not be just right for you."

"What does that mean?" I asked, feeling the now familiar sense of panic returning.

"Well, there's one other pill I want to try with this one. The two of them together might have a better effect," he said, scrawling on his prescription pad.

"'Might?'" I asked. "What do you mean, 'might'? What if this doesn't work?"

"If this doesn't work, we'll put you on insulin," he told me matter-of-factly.

"Insulin? I don't think I want to take insulin," I ventured naively, as if I had some other alternative.

"Let's not get ahead of ourselves," he said, not wanting to have a premature discussion about insulin therapy. "Start on these other pills today, keep up with your glucose testing, and make an appointment to come back in on Friday."

I took the additional pills as instructed and returned to the doctor on schedule three days later with no better glucose levels to report. I knew what he was going to tell me. He was going to tell me I had Type 1 diabetes. I was going to have to start giving myself injections of insulin.

"So I have to give myself shots?" I asked, my voice quaking.

"Yes, I'll explain that," the doctor responded.

"I know this is a silly question, but I have to ask," I laughed nervously and tried to sound as if I were kidding. "Isn't there some other way to take insulin? I mean, can't I just swallow it or put it in my food or something? I suppose they've tried that, and it doesn't work?" I was not kidding. I was grasping at straws.

"As of yet, there's no other way. There's an inhalable form of insulin that's in clinical studies now, but that's still a few years off. Right now, injections are the only way."

The doctor did this for a living. Every day, for the past thirty-five years or so, he had treated patients who gave themselves daily injections of insulin in order to survive. This was routine for him. This was not routine for me. This was terrifying for me.

"I don't know if I can do it," I stammered.

The doctor regarded me sympathetically. "You can do it. Nobody likes to hear that they have to start taking insulin. But you can do it. You'll have it figured out in no time."

"Will it definitely work?" I asked. I wanted to know if there was a possibility that I could go through this ordeal and then find out that the insulin, like the pills, did not work.

"Oh, it will work," he smiled assuredly. "It always works."

He explained that I would be taking two different types of insulin: a long-acting form and a short-acting form. It was news to me that there were different types of insulin. I would have guessed that insulin is insulin is insulin. But in fact they're absorbed at different rates, and they remain active in the body for different periods of time.

The long-acting insulin that was available when I was diagnosed started working within a few hours after injection, peaked gradually about nine to twelve hours after injection, and wore off within about twenty-four hours. This would give me a baseline level of glucose control but would not be sufficient to cover spikes in glucose levels that occur after eating. For those short-term increases in glucose levels, there was short-acting insulin. When I started taking insulin, the shortest-acting insulin available started working within thirty to sixty minutes after injection, peaked in one to three hours, and wore off five to seven hours later.

The doctor explained that correctly timing the "peak" of insulin would be crucial to successfully managing insulin therapy. When insulin peaks, it is working its hardest to get the glucose from the carbohydrates into your cells. Ideally, the peak of the insulin should coincide with the time when carbohydrates from a meal are getting into your bloodstream. Miscalculate the peak, and you could end up with a glucose level that is too high (if the insulin peaks early and is no longer available to cover the carbohydrates that you have consumed), or you could end up with a glucose level that is too low (if the carbohydrates you have consumed are not sufficient to offset the peaking insulin).

So the irony of insulin therapy is that its purpose is to counteract high blood sugar, but if the peak of the insulin is not timed correctly, it can cause low blood sugar. Low blood sugar is a different, and more immediately dangerous, aspect of being on insulin.

After walking me through Insulin Training 101, the doctor gave me two little glass vials. One vial was full of a clear liquid; this was the short-acting insulin. The other vial was full of a liquid that was a bit murky and appeared to have settled at the bottom of the vial; this was the long-acting insulin. The long-acting insulin needed to be mixed before it was injected. The doctor showed me the technique for rolling the vial of insulin between my hands until the particles that had settled at the bottom of the vial had turned the mixture cloudy.

Then he explained to me how to draw the insulin out of the vial and into a syringe and then to give myself a shot. First, use an alcohol pad to clean the spot on your body where you will give the injection. The injection is administered subcutaneously, which means it goes under the skin, not into the blood stream. The most common injection sites are the abdomen, the upper arm, the thigh, and the buttocks.

Once you have chosen and sterilized the injection site, wipe the top of the vial of insulin with the alcohol pad. If you are using long-acting insulin, roll the vial in your hands to mix it. Pull the plunger back into the syringe, drawing in air until the plunger reaches the mark on the syringe for the number of units that you will inject. Insert the needle tip of the syringe into the vial of insulin and inject the air into the vial.

Next, holding the needle still in the vial (and paying no mind to your trembling hands), invert the vial so that it is upside down. Pull back the plunger again, as you did initially to fill it with air, but this time the magic fluid will fill the syringe as the plunger is pulled back. Watch for air bubbles as you fill the syringe. If there are bubbles, rap the syringe sharply to knock them out. I pictured myself sitting on an examination table in a doctor's office as a child, watching as a nurse tapped an inverted syringe and squirted some fluid from the syringe into the air before giving me a vaccination. The same general principle was at work here, with the significant difference being that I, rather than a nurse, would be responsible for the execution.

"So that's pretty much it," the doctor concluded.

"I don't know if I got all of that," I responded. In truth, my concentration had started to fade before he even completed the discussion of the different types of insulin. "Do you have this written down somewhere? Something that I can bring home with me?"

"Oh yes, yes, of course we do. I'll be sending you off with a whole new set of brochures. They'll explain it all. This was just an overview."

"So when do I take my first shot?" I asked hesitantly. I was still holding out hope that he would remember that there was one other possible treatment that he had forgotten to try on me. I was waiting for him to say, *Wait a minute. You know, I don't think you have to do this after all. I think something else might work for you.* It was his last chance to call off the shots.

"Tomorrow. You should take your first shot about a half hour before you eat breakfast tomorrow." So this was it. He was not going to suggest something else. This was really it.

"Okay then," I said halfheartedly. No, not even halfheartedly. My heart was not in this one at all. My heart was nowhere to be found.

He saw my dismay. "If you like, you can do a shot here, right now. I wanted to wait until the morning for you to start on the long-acting, but you could take a short-acting shot here." He was trying to help me out.

"Uh, well, no. I think I'll wait. I'll do it in the morning, like you said. I'll do it then."

"You can practice on an orange," he said.

"I beg your pardon?" I asked, picturing myself withdrawing juice from an orange into a syringe.

Apparently I had the vision backward for the doctor explained that it was not the withdrawal but rather the injection that was practiced on an orange. *Why on earth would I practice an injection on an orange?* I thought to myself. I was no scientist, but the last time I checked, an orange feels no pain. What was the point of practicing an injection on a piece of fruit that feels no pain?

*   *   *

"What's the matter with Amy?" Willie, Paul's younger son, asked. We had spared Willie and his older brother, Ned, the drama of the past week. Now that I was going to start taking insulin, though, we needed to let them know what was going on.

"We wanted to talk to you guys about that," Paul began. We were all in the living room. Paul and I were side by side on the couch; Ned and Willie were wrestling on the floor.

"I want to tell them. Let me tell them," I said. Adopting what I thought was a tone appropriate for boys ages four and seven, I said, "Well, I wasn't feeling very well, and so I went to the doctor, and the doctor told me that I have something called diabetes. Have you guys ever heard of that?"

They paused to consider the question. Then four-year-old Willie, the budding wordsmith, said, "Hey, maybe you're going to die. Get it? *Die*-betes?"

"Willie, don't say that!" Ned delivered a hard whack to Willie's arm.

Ned looked at Paul. "That's not true," he said. "She's not going to die, is she, Dad?"

"No," Paul and I responded as one.

"Of course not. That's the silliest thing I've ever heard," I said to the boys.

"But you look so sad," Ned said. "Why are you sad if you're not going to die?"

"I'm not sad," I lied, "but I am nervous." Now I was telling the truth. "I'm nervous because I have to give myself shots every day. And I'm scared that the shots are going to hurt. That's all. I do the first one tomorrow morning."

The boys squealed and shrieked at the delightfully gruesome thought of me having to give myself a shot. "Gross. Oh my gosh— that's gonna hurt." And then they asked a question that surprised me: "Can we watch?"

"Can you watch?" I didn't know what to say.

"Yeah, can we watch you do your shot tomorrow?" They stared at me in eager anticipation.

Paul tried to intercede. "Guys, come on. Amy might want some privacy."

What the hell, I thought to myself. *The more the merrier.* "Sure, you can watch."

"Yay," they shouted. And then they were off, Willie chanting, "Di-a-be-tes, di-a-be-tes," to the tune of *Frère Jacques*, as they headed to their playroom upstairs. We had held their attention for as long as humanly possible

The next day, a Saturday, dawned hot and humid again. I had not slept well the night before. I had been alone at my apartment that night, and in addition to now being freaked out about being alone, I was also freaked out about injecting that first shot of insulin. I didn't know how I was going to make myself do it. I didn't know how I was going to force myself to stick a needle under my skin, hold it in place, and depress the plunger to force out the insulin. The thought of it nearly paralyzed me. But I pushed through, got into my car, and drove over to Paul's home.

Sticking a needle into your own body isn't an intuitive act. From the time we're toddlers, we're taught to point sharp objects away from us. Walk with scissors pointing down. Don't run with a pencil in your hand. Pass a knife by the handle, not blade first. If you find a needle, a pin, a piece of broken glass, don't touch it. Fortunately for most of us, our only experiences with shots were the vaccinations we received as young children. The anticipation of those shots was dreadful, and often the reality was even more painful than we had feared.

So at first it seems incomprehensible to learn that you must have injections every day in order to survive. It is more baffling still to learn that you have to administer them yourself. When you first hear the news, the question of how many injections doesn't even occur to you. The fact that you have to give yourself even one shot is stunning enough. What you don't know at that point, but what you will learn, is that if you can do it once, you can do it a thousand times. And if you have Type 1 diabetes, you will do it a thousand times, perhaps just during your first year with the disease.

Now, having given myself more than ten thousand injections, I can say that there has been no injection worse than that first one. No matter how uncomfortable some of them were, and no matter how many times I accidentally drew blood, and no matter how many times I had to push the needle harder than I would have liked, feeling and hearing it pop through each layer of bruised tissue, that first shot I gave myself was without a doubt the worst. My first shot was a pure triumph of will.

I sat down on the edge of Paul's bed. He stood beside me, poised as if to rescue me from something. Ned and Willie were on the floor in front of me, on their knees, inching closer and closer to try to get the best view.

It actually helped to have Paul and the boys watching. I had to pretend to be brave. I didn't have to pretend for Paul—I had given up on that the day of my diagnosis. But I did have to pretend for the boys. I didn't want them to know how scared I was.

"Stay back. Don't touch her," Paul cautioned the boys.

"Listen to your dad, guys. Don't touch me. I have to be really still," I told them. They inched back a little. "That's good. You're good right there." I wiped a patch of skin on the front of my thigh with an alcohol swab. I rolled the vial of insulin between my hands until the liquid was cloudy. I withdrew the prescribed amount into the syringe. I pinched the skin of my thigh into a little mound. I pressed the needle against the crest of the pinched skin, to feel how sharp it was. It was very sharp.

I looked at Paul. "I don't think I can do this." So much for my fake bravery.

"You can do it, baby," Paul said, placing a hand on my shoulder. "Come on, you can do it. You have to do it." The boys were holding their breath, silent with anticipation.

And then I did it. I pushed the needle through my skin. The boys squirmed and squealed with delight, "She's doing it. Oh my gosh, she's actually doing it." I pushed the plunger down to force out the insulin. I withdrew the needle at a bad angle, not the same angle at which I had inserted it, and felt a burning sensation where I had withdrawn it.

Paul leaned down to hug me "You did it, baby," he whispered into my ear. "You did it."

"Did it hurt? Did it hurt?" the boys wanted to know.

"Not really," I said truthfully. "It just felt weird, and now it kind of stings, but it didn't really hurt like I thought it was going to."

"Then why are you crying?" Ned asked.

"Am I crying?" I said, reaching up to touch my cheek and finding to my surprise that it was wet. "Wow, I didn't even notice. I guess it's just the excitement of it all." I stood up from the bed and made a move to deflect the attention away from me. "Okay, show's over. Nothing more to see here, folks, move on out," I teased as I ushered Paul and the boys out of the room.

Why had I been crying? I wondered. The shot really had not caused me enough physical pain to induce tears. I shrugged off the episode, chalking it up to emotional exhaustion. Looking back now at the months that followed, and at the period of adjustment that came with learning to live as a person with insulin-dependent diabetes, I know that I was crying because I was beginning to mourn. I was beginning to mourn the loss of my old life, a life that did not require syringes, insulin, and glucose meters.

*   *   *

For the rest of that summer, I adjusted reluctantly to my new life, amazed at how difficult it was. I read as much as I could about diabetes, but this was 1996. There was no webmd; there was no Wikipedia; there was no American Diabetes Association home page. There was no central place to find information easily. Most of my reading was in books, in pamphlets, and in journal or magazine articles.

After a time, the information became repetitive. The word "survive" cropped up in my reading far more often than I would have liked, as in "Type 1 diabetics must take daily injections of insulin in order to survive." Survive is such a severe word, so irreversible in its consequences. You survive, or you don't. It's a one-shot deal. There are no degrees of survival.

I didn't want to be subject to a treatment for which survival was the touchstone. I wanted desperately to have a less dramatic course of treatment. I wanted to take a medicine that was prescribed to perform some benign function such as "alleviate symptoms of discomfort," or use a medicine that had gentle side effects such as "may cause drowsiness." And I know I could have lived with the standard: "Do not operate heavy machinery after taking this medication." But I wasn't sure how to live under this new regime where survival was the benchmark.

So I read. I read, and I read, and I read. I just knew that if I searched hard enough, I would eventually come across the little hook that my doctors and all the researchers to date had missed. I would come across a footnote in an article that explained why I, Amy Fitzgerald, who had weathered so many challenges already in her life, who was now so happy, who had so much to look forward to, did not really have to give herself shots of insulin every day in order to survive. I was going to find the magic information in the small print that could rescue me from the life that other insulin-dependent diabetics were destined to live. I'm still searching for that footnote.

It is a gradual but nonetheless suffocating process to realize what it means to live with a chronic health condition. After I had been giving myself injections of insulin for a week, two weeks, one month, I thought I should be able to stop. Enough already; I got it. I had done the shots, my glucose levels were very often in the green zone. I was with the program. So shouldn't I be able to stop at some point? But that is not what chronic means. Chronic does not let you stop.

In my quest to find some objective meaning to pin on my situation, I looked up the word "chronic" in the dictionary. And there it was, the definition I had been searching for: *always present; constantly vexing.* I couldn't have said it better myself. However, I didn't understand then what "always" means. I understand now. Always means you don't get to stop your treatment—ever. Always means you don't get to forget about your condition—ever. Always means every day, every night, every hour, every meal, every nap, every walk, every meeting, every trip to the grocery store, every finger prick. Always is relentless. And insulin therapy is vexing. Always.

7

"*Wow, that's bad,*" *my brother* said when he heard about my diagnosis. "Are you still going to go to law school?" It's always surprising what people will say to me.

"Yes, of course I am," I answered. "I thought I might not throw in the towel just yet."

As it turned out, starting law school a few months after I started on insulin was a good thing. There's nothing like fear of the Socratic method to take your mind off your other problems.

I established a routine when I started law school. Shortly after waking up, I would pad bleary-eyed into the bathroom, prick my finger, and do my first glucose test of the day (test #1). I would then shuffle to the fridge, where I stored my insulin, remove the vial of long-acting insulin, roll it between my hands to mix it, and do my first shot of the day. The long-acting insulin would begin to act within a couple of hours and so should cover the breakfast that I would eat about an hour after injecting that first shot. I would then shower, get dressed, eat breakfast, and walk with a fifteen-to-twenty-pound backpack for about half a mile to the metro station. I would take that into Washington, D.C., and then have about another quarter of a mile to walk from the metro station to my law school.

When I arrived at school, I would head first thing into the ladies' room, sling off my backpack in one of the cramped stalls, get out my glucose meter, find a place to balance it—lap, top of backpack, or last and least favorite, atop the toilet paper dispenser—and do another glucose test (test #2). With this second test, I needed to know how the walk from home to the metro and the walk from the metro to law

68

school had affected my glucose level. Typically, exercise lowers your glucose level, and on some days walking with my heavy backpack would cause my glucose level to fall too low. After seeing the results of my second glucose test of the day, and determining whether or not I needed to eat a snack to boost my glucose level, I would go to the library and do some reading before my classes started.

I loved to spend an hour or two every morning studying in the grand main reading room of the law school library. It was a quint-essential reading room: rich burgundy carpet; row after row of long, sturdy mahogany reading tables; low lighting punctuated every few feet with bursts of brightness from brass lamps on the reading tables; and a heavy, almost audible hum of silence. It's the kind of room in which the law is meant to be studied.

When it was time to leave the library and head to class, I would prick my finger again (test #3). If there was no one nearby who would notice the beep of my glucose meter, I would place it in my lap and do the test right there. If people were nearby, though, I wouldn't want to draw attention to myself, so I would steal away to a bathroom stall. The purpose of this third glucose test of the day was to make sure that I was not heading into a low when I went into class. My classes were typically either forty-five or ninety minutes long. Based on my pre-class glucose level, I would have a good idea of whether I needed a snack to maintain my glucose level during class. After class, I would prick my finger again (test #4) and give myself an injection of short-acting insulin before eating lunch. The long-acting insulin I had taken before breakfast would not cover my lunch carbohydrates, so I had to give myself a dose of short-acting insulin before lunch (shot #2). I then would eat lunch and go to my afternoon class or classes. After classes ended, I would duck into a bathroom stall again to prick my finger before pulling on my backpack and setting off on the quarter-mile walk back to the metro (test #5).

At the other end of my metro commute, I would do the half-mile walk home. Shortly after getting home, I would do another glucose test (test #6) to see if I needed a snack before dinner. As with the morning walks during my commute to the metro, the evening walks might have brought my glucose level down too low.

After spending some time organizing my notes from classes that day and getting myself organized for the next day, I would cook myself a simple dinner. Before dinner I would do another glucose test (test #7). If my pre-dinner glucose level was within the normal range, I would not need to take another shot of short-acting insulin, for the long-acting insulin I had taken at breakfast would be peaking about the time I ate dinner. If my glucose level was high before dinner, I might give myself a small dose of short-acting insulin (which would be shot #3) to bring my glucose level back into the green zone. Before going to bed I would test my glucose level one more time (test #8).

So there it was: eight glucose tests and three shots of insulin on a good day. And most days were not good days. Most days were days when I needed to do more tests because I wanted to exercise, or I was going to drive somewhere, or I felt low and needed to check.

I am fortunate enough to have medical insurance that covers most of the costs of my glucose testing, and more fortunate still to have the financial means to cover out-of-pocket costs for glucose-testing supplies when my prescription for them has run out. Glucose test strips are a tremendous expense. When I was diagnosed, the cost of a vial of fifty test strips was $34.99, or about seventy cents per strip. Multiply this by eight tests per day, and the cost was $5.60 per day, on a good day, for keeping up my with my glucose tests. That is almost $40 per week—over $2,000 per year. Not surprisingly, the cost of test strips has gone up over the years. The last vial of fifty that I bought cost $61.99. That's $1.24 per strip, $9.91 per day, $69.43 per week, $3,610 per year. The costs pile up exponentially.

These are real costs that someone pays. In my case that someone, for the most part, is my medical insurance company. My endocrinologist writes a prescription for me for three months' worth of test strips at a time and prescribes ten tests per day. Because I usually end up testing more than ten times a day, I often run out of test strips a week or two before my three-month prescription is eligible for renewal. When this happens, I go out-of-pocket and spend the $100 or so required to keep me in test strips until I can renew my prescription.

As difficult as this disease is to manage, I can't imagine trying to do it without comprehensive medical insurance and without ample quantities of my own funds to fall back on. I'm lucky to be in this position. Each time I get a new shipment of three months' worth of test strips, and each time I have to pay for my own test strips between prescriptions, I'm conscious of the fact that there are many others with my disease who are not so lucky. I don't know how they do it.

8

Let me explain a bit more about low glucose levels, which I have mentioned a few times. Of course, to a degree, a person with diabetes wants her glucose levels to be low. After all, high glucose levels, the hallmark of diabetes, are what cause the dreadful, long-term complications of diabetes. So, to an extent, low glucose levels are a good thing. But they're only a good thing if they don't fall too low.

A glucose level that's too low poses serious and immediate risks that need to be addressed in a matter of minutes. Untreated, a low glucose level can cause unconsciousness, seizures, and, in rare and extreme cases, even death. Rare and extreme, yes, but an insulin-dependent diabetic does not have to read these possible outcomes more than once to forever fear lows.

The greatest and most cruel irony of managing Type 1 diabetes is that insulin, the substance that you need to survive—the only thing on earth that will bring your high glucose levels back to the normal range—can also harm you. The tighter you try to manage your disease (that is, the more you try to keep your glucose levels in the normal range), the more likely you are to suffer lows. And here we find ourselves again in the definition of "chronic": Insulin therapy is constantly vexing.

Generally, a low (or, to use the technical term, "hypoglycemia") is considered to be a glucose level below 70. If you have diabetes and you are lucky, you have a good internal early warning system. Perhaps when your glucose level starts falling into the 70s, or maybe even the 80s, you feel one or more of the telltale symptoms of a low. Maybe you start to feel a little nervous, or a little irritable, or a little impatient. Or maybe you start to perspire, your heart flutters and pounds, your hands tremble, and you feel weak. Or maybe you feel a sudden and overwhelming fatigue, a desire to just crumple where you are, close your eyes, and let the exhaustion overwhelm you.

The trick to managing a low is to feel it coming on and to cut it off at the pass by eating or drinking some form of glucose that gets into the bloodstream quickly. Fruit juice, milk, and soda are good for these purposes, as are honey, sugar cubes, and glucose pills (sugar tablets that are available over the counter). To counteract a low, you ingest one of these or some other form of fast-acting sugar—usually about fifteen grams of carbohydrates is the recommended amount—and then wait ten to fifteen minutes before doing a glucose test to see whether your glucose level is coming up. Depending on how severe the low is and what particular symptoms are present, that can be a very long ten to fifteen minutes. If your glucose level has not come up to an acceptable level in that time, you take some more sugar and try again with a glucose test ten to fifteen minutes later. And so on, until your glucose level has come up sufficiently.

When I'm getting too low, there's one symptom I can always count on: confusion. It's a strange and intense kind of confusion—a kind of confusion that literally can cause me to close my eyes, furrow my brow, and try to understand what's happening all around me. It's not the kind of confusion that you experience when you don't understand a math problem or when you can't think of the right word to complete a crossword puzzle. It's the kind of confusion that doesn't let you process a thought from start to finish. Thoughts form, balloon up, then burst and drift away into thin air. There's no closure to any thought. There's no comprehension. It's a feeling of being utterly lost and not knowing how to get from point A to point B.

The first severe low I ever suffered was during the summer a year after my diagnosis. I had just completed my first year of law school and was working as a summer associate at a law firm in Washington, D.C. The firm had the practice, as many do, of taking summer associates out every day for lavish lunches. Most days I dined in the most trendy lunch spots in the city. On this particular day, however, I did not have lunch plans with anyone from the firm. It was a rare day when I was going out alone to pick up lunch and bring it back to my office to eat, the way the rest of the world did. It was actually a relief to be on my own and not have to perform during what amounted to a daily job interview over lunch.

I was headed to a little deli near my office that had my favorite sandwich—tomato, mozzarella, and basil on grilled bread. I knew its name and its ingredients by heart. Now that I had my insulin doses figured out and knew how to use short-acting insulin to cover a high-carb meal like a grilled sandwich, I could eat it to my heart's content—as long as I covered it with the right amount of insulin.

Before leaving the office, I checked my glucose level: 129. Perfect. Not too high, not too low. It was precisely in the range I wanted to see. Although a glucose level of 129 would be bad news for someone who does not have diabetes, but it's good news for an insulin-dependent diabetic who wants to walk to a restaurant and pick up lunch. My last injection of insulin had been about five and a half hours before, and that had been the long-acting dose I took before I ate breakfast. That insulin was still active, it wasn't peaking yet, and so a glucose level of 129 should have been more than enough to get me through the next half hour or so until I got back to the office with my sandwich.

I packed up my glucose meter and put it in my purse, double-checked my supply of glucose pills (ever cautious, ever nervous, better safe than sorry), and headed out of the office. It was a July day, characterized by the three Hs that weathermen in Washington, D.C., recite nightly during the summer forecasts: hazy, hot, and humid. In fact, it was beyond humid. The air itself felt thick and damp. It also looked as though it might rain at any moment. I thought briefly about going back inside to get an umbrella but decided against it. I really was happy to have some time alone during my lunch break. I also didn't want to risk a return to the building where I might encounter some well-intentioned attorney who would realize that I didn't have lunch plans and who might insist on saving me from my solitude.

My first stop was at a cash machine about a block away. Unbelievably, there was no line. I made a withdrawal and continued toward the restaurant. When I arrived, it was packed. Evidently there had been no line at the bank because every person in a ten-block radius had chosen my restaurant for lunch. I took my place in the queue, scanned the menu that was on the wall, found the entry for the sandwich that I knew by heart, and settled in for a long wait.

Minutes slogged by, and I shuffled forward gradually toward a gruff, older man, who was taking the orders. The ordering process seemed chaotic: You had to place your order in response to his command—"Order, please." The commander then gave you a slip of paper with the name of the item you ordered printed on it, which you took to the cashier. After paying, you were herded into a holding area until your order number (printed on your receipt) was called out, at which time you picked up your order.

All of the other customers at the restaurant seemed to know the ropes, but I found the whole ordering process to be very confusing and just a bit intimidating. A misstep at any point along the ordering chain would cause needless delay and risk annoying either the commander or the cashier or both and frustrating the veteran patrons who were in line behind me. I decided to rehearse my order in my head so that I would be ready when called on. I knew very well what I had come here to get. It was the... the.... What was it? I could not think of it. I couldn't think of my favorite sandwich. I looked up at the menu to see if that would trigger my memory, but I didn't see what I wanted. All I saw were letters. Letters and numbers.

"Order, please," I heard someone saying. I was still peering at the menu, trying to make some sense of it. The letters and numbers were right there on the menu board, but I couldn't comprehend them.

"Order, please," I heard again.

"Miss, it's your turn," the person behind me said and tapped my shoulder lightly.

"My turn?" I asked, not understanding what he was telling me. "I'm not sure..." My voice trailed off.

"It's your turn to order," the person explained.

"Are you going to order?" the commander asked, "because if you're not, you need to get out of line." Why were these people talking to me? What did they want me to do?

I wasn't sure what to do. I thought I should prick my finger, but I couldn't figure out how to do a glucose test there in the line, without a surface on which to rest my glucose meter and without drawing curious stares.

"Do you have a bathroom?" I asked the commander.

"Bathroom's over there," he said, waving his arm in the general direction of a door across the room. "Are you gonna order?"

"Um, no.... No, I don't think so," I muttered as I turned to head toward the bathroom. My legs felt wobbly, and I had the impression that all eyes in the restaurant were on me as I crossed the room. I went into the bathroom, locked the door, situated my glucose meter on the counter by the sink, and pricked my finger. My heart was racing. Streams of sweat trickled down the sides of my face, and beneath my shirt my chest was wet with perspiration. The wetness made me cold in the air-conditioned bathroom. I saw myself in the mirror. My face was white, my eyes wide and vacant.

The beep of my glucose meter reminded me that I needed to look at the screen to see what my glucose level was. The number I saw was way too low: 48. I dug around in my purse for my glucose pills, found the bottle, and dumped several into my hand. I tried to count them but I couldn't. I shoved a handful of the big, chalky pills into my mouth and chewed laboriously. Glucose pills have the consistency of sweet tarts or baby aspirin, many times the size, and it takes a bit of jaw power to get them going.

Then all I could do was wait for the glucose pills to take effect. But wait where? I couldn't stay in the bathroom. At least I knew that. Maybe I could find a table in the restaurant, sit down, and wait there. I left the bathroom and re-entered the chaos of the restaurant. I wove through the dining room, trying to find a place to sit, but every table was occupied. I thought of asking someone if I could sit at her table for a few minutes, but I didn't think I could explain myself. I decided instead to walk back to my office.

I left the restaurant and headed off in what I believed to be the direction of my office. I walked until I got to the corner of the next block. There was one sign that said "20th" and one sign that said "NEW HAMPSHIRE." More numbers and letters. I knew these were symbols that I had seen before. I knew they were supposed to mean something to me, but I couldn't for the life of me figure out what it was. I tried to think of where my office was. New Hampshire looked familiar, but I was not sure about the 20th. I didn't know which way to go. And I was so tired. I was exhausted. My legs felt as if they wouldn't support me much longer.

I sat down on a bench near the street corner and stared up at the numbers 2 and 0 on the street sign. Were those my numbers? The rain that I had anticipated when I left the office started to fall lightly. I reached into my purse for a few more glucose pills, found them, and worked them into my mouth. I looked down at my MedicAlert bracelet. I had long since given up the DIABETES plaque bracelet that I had bought at the drugstore the evening of my diagnosis, and now wore a MedicAlert bracelet that linked me to my individual health information. I thought about walking into a building or stopping a passerby, showing someone my bracelet, and saying, "I need help." But even lost in my hypoglycemic confusion, I knew there was nothing anyone could do to help. I knew that in the time it would take to make someone understand what was wrong with me, I could get better. The glucose pills might kick in anytime. I had eaten my first round in the bathroom at the restaurant and chewed the second round just moments ago. All I could do was wait—sit in the rain, stare vacantly, and wait.

In time, the glucose from the pills that I had eaten began to make its way into my bloodstream. The vacant feeling began to leave me and in its place descended a heavy feeling of self-consciousness. I became aware that I was sitting on an unsheltered bench on a street corner during a light rain. I felt overwhelmingly sad at my predicament but no longer so disoriented. I stood up and walked to the corner. I knew where I was. My office was half a block away on New Hampshire Avenue. I could see it easily from the intersection that had confounded me just minutes before. In the rain I returned to the bench, sat down, and pricked my finger. 87. I was going to be okay. My glucose level was coming up. I could find my way back to the office.

This one severe low, suffered when I was alone, was all it took to make me very afraid of lows. The fact that it had come on without much warning, when I had left the office with what should have been a high-enough glucose level not thirty minutes earlier, made it all the more troubling. This experience left me with the sense that a low can get me at any time, and without much warning: while I'm sleeping; while I'm taking a walk; while I'm leading a meeting; while I'm watching a school production; while I'm running errands.

Lows are the episodes that give insulin-dependent diabetics a bad name. They're what lead people to believe that we're moody, temperamental, and unpredictable. I'm not sure whether I was aware that such a stereotype existed until the first time that I unwittingly found myself on the receiving end of an ugly comment about people who have diabetes. This happened during the same summer I suffered the traumatic low in the rain outside the deli.

I was meeting with a young lawyer with whom I was working on a project. We were about to call the client to get further direction on our assignment, and he was giving me some background information to help set the stage for our client call. He briefed me on the nature of the client's business, the personalities involved, and who would likely be most vocal on the call. As he was explaining his take on the personalities, he singled out one man for special mention: "Now we have to watch out for him," he cautioned. "He's your typically temperamental diabetic," and with that he continued to scroll through the list of names of who would be on the call.

I was stunned. I didn't hear the next few sentences he said. His lips were moving, his arms were gesturing, and his face was expressive, but I couldn't hear a word he said. His ugly words kept repeating themselves in my head: *Your typically temperamental diabetic....* How dare he say such a thing?

When I regained my senses and rejoined the conversation, I did something that I've been ashamed of ever since: I let his comment go. I didn't speak up in defense of people with diabetes. I didn't point out that lots of people are temperamental, whether or not they have diabetes. I didn't tell him that his comment was unfair, unjustified, ill-informed, and hurtful. Why didn't I?

9

I replayed that scene many times in my head during the months that followed. My imaginary, replayed version of the scene came out quite differently. In response to his comment, I said in a menacing tone, rising from my chair, "Excuse me, but *I* am a typically temperamental diabetic."

In my imaginary scene he straightened in his chair and looked nervous as I walked around his desk to meet him. He realized, too late, that he had pissed off the wrong person with diabetes. As I delivered my powerful fist into his jaw, I said calmly, "And I *hate* being called temperamental." Then I turned neatly, walked back across the office, flipped over the chair that I had been sitting in, ripped open the door, and left it swinging wide on its hinges after my exit, exposing the wounded bigot to the gasping crowd that had gathered outside his office door.

I knew this version was a little Dirty Harry-ish and not something close to what I would ever do in real life, but it was fun to think about. And it was easier to think about than trying to unpack the real reasons why I hadn't spoken up. One reason was that my response might have proven the stereotype that he already believed. My response wouldn't have involved fisticuffs or chairs toppling, but it would have involved an anger that would have been hard to mask, and a quaking voice that would have betrayed the stable demeanor I would have hoped to convey. More than likely it would have been temperamental. My reaction would have had nothing to do with the fact that I had diabetes, of course, but it would have cemented his ill-founded views.

Another reason I didn't respond was that I didn't want to pub-licly claim ownership of my disease. I didn't want the label. I didn't want to be the summer associate who had diabetes. Like it or not, having a disease labels you. It tells people one specific thing about you. It doesn't tell them anything else, just that one thing. But that one thing can be enough to let them think that they know who you are or why you are how you are, simply by identifying one of your least fortunate traits—an immutable health condition.

A friend of mine had breast cancer, early stage, completely recov-erable and survivable. She took medical leave from her job in order to be treated and to have surgery. She told no one about her condi-tion except for me and a handful of close friends. Our many other friends and colleagues were concerned, asking about her health and the reasons for her absence, but she wouldn't tell them.

"I don't want to be the woman with breast cancer," she said to me.

"But you wouldn't be," I assured her. "People just want to know so they can help you. So they know how you are. Everyone knows you are you. No one's going to start referring to you as the woman with breast cancer."

"You're wrong, Amy. They will." To prove her point, she said, "How about Mary Smith? Do you know Mary Smith?"

Before I could catch myself, I answered, "Oh, you mean the woman in tax, the one who had breast cancer?" And there I was, referring to a human being by her disease. What I didn't want for myself I had inflicted on someone else.

Sometimes I don't even know how to tell someone that I have this disease. When I do say, "I have diabetes,"— a revelation that often leads to the presumption that I have Type 2, which is the type most people have heard about. I try never to compare diseases, either within the diabetes world or outside it. Who's to say whether someone who has Type 2 has it easier than someone who has Type 1? Or whether someone who has Type 1 has it easier than someone who has some other disease? It's a losing game to compare miseries, to try to prove that someone else has it easier than you do.

Nevertheless, when I name my disease to the uninformed, I am relieved that I don't have to claim it as Type 2, which receives a heavy dose of judgment from the outside world. I can't think of another disease that is seen as frequently in headlines. Most of the stories behind the headlines suggest that the people who have Type 2 diabetes brought it on themselves with poor eating habits and a sedentary lifestyle. They lay on an additional level of guilt by reminding the affected that at the current rate of incidence, people who have Type 2 diabetes will put a tremendous strain on the healthcare system.

They don't mention that Type 2 diabetes is a complicated disease with a number of possible causes. They don't mention that genetics plays a large role in Type 2 diabetes, regardless of lifestyle choices. They make the occurrence of Type 2 diabetes sound like a causal effect that results only from poor lifestyle choices, while in fact lifestyle choices may be more a correlative than a causative factor.

But whatever the cause of Type 2 diabetes, the afflicted are made to feel that they could have avoided it altogether with smarter choices. With the possible exceptions of lung cancer for a smoker or cirrhosis of the liver for an alcoholic, I can't think of another illness that provokes the self-righteous sentiment that the recipients got what they asked for: *If you hadn't been sitting around on the couch all day, drinking soda and eating fast food, while the healthier among us were going to yoga and eating five servings of vegetables a day, you wouldn't have gotten yourself into this mess.*

When some people have erroneously concluded that I suffer from Type 2 diabetes, they have actually offered comments like, "Really? Can't you go on a diet or something?" or "Don't you exercise?" I'm glad I don't have to deal with that prejudice. I'm glad that for all the misery that comes with my type of this disease, I don't have to suffer with the guilt of being made to feel that I could have prevented it, and defending myself against the questions of the uninformed.

So to distinguish myself from the Type 2s, sometimes I say I have juvenile diabetes. Many people know that's the "other kind," the bad kind, as people have also remarked to me before. But that designation misses the mark as well, because so many people believe that juvenile diabetes is a disease of childhood. "Don't you outgrow that?" I was asked just recently.

When I decide to tell, when I decide to make public this most private condition, I tend to say that I have Type 1 diabetes. And then the questions start: *Which kind is that? Should you be eating that if you have diabetes? Are you going to faint or start talking nonsense?* This latter comment came from a work colleague, a brilliant lawyer, who was not sure what to do with me when I told him I would need to step out of an all-day negotiation periodically to check my glucose level.

I know that when I tell, I will be labeled. But whatever label others might put on me, whatever misconceptions come along with bearing the label of this disease that has just one name but several different forms, there can be no label harsher than the one I put on myself: failure.

At the most basic level, my body has failed me. My immune system destroys what I need to stay alive. It kills the insulin-producing beta cells in my pancreas. It isn't just the diabetes: I have, since my diagnosis of diabetes, developed rheumatoid arthritis, a condition in which my immune system destroys what my joints need to stay functional. The joints in my hands and feet swell and ache wrenchingly. Simply fastening a button can be a sweat-inducing terror some days. My body, for some reason, is not that interested in keeping me going. In fact, it tries to do just the opposite. It tries to shut me down. I am, however, strongly interested in keeping myself going. I don't want to be shut down. But it is a battle against this hateful immune system of mine each and every day.

It isn't just my body that fails me—I fail myself. I fail to control my diabetes in the very tight manner that we, the royal "we" who have diabetes in this day and age, are told we should be able to do. We have the tools to manage our disease far more effectively than would ever have been possible, or even imaginable, twenty-five years ago. We have portable glucose monitors and continuous glucose monitors. We have long-acting insulin, short-acting insulin, and insulin pumps. We have super-fine-tipped syringes, syringe pens, everything we need to make our shots less painful. We have, in theory, everything at our disposal that our doctors and the medical-device companies and pharmaceutical companies tell us should enable us to control our disease. Yet control eludes us. Control eludes me. And when control eludes me, I am a failure.

I am a failure when a family hike is cut short because what should have been a high-enough glucose level won't get me to the top of the mountain, and my family refuses to leave me behind. I am a failure when I am reduced to begging a jar of pureed baby food from a family walking across the Golden Gate Bridge, when what should have been an ample stock of glucose pills has run out and I have no hope of making it across the bridge, nor of turning around and making it back. I am a failure when I gobble down a granola bar before a meeting and don't take any insulin, jacking my glucose level far too high so I don't have to worry about a low for the next few hours. I am a failure when my quarterly blood tests show that I should be able to do better. When it comes to having diabetes, I fail again and again and again.

If I tell someone the name of my disease, if I tell them my label, will they be able to read the subtext? Will they know, just by my acknowledgment of my disease, that I am failing at it? Can they see that far into me, to know how bearing this label feels to me? Perhaps that's why I didn't respond to the lawyer's comment about temperamental diabetics. Maybe my response would have proved too much, would have given too much insight into how I feel about who I am with this disease.

Control is the buzzword for the person with diabetes. We are asked, and we ask ourselves, time and again, whether we are in control.

That is so intrusive a notion that it reaches far beyond the mere status of a disease. Would I ever ask this question of a person who does not have diabetes? Would I ever ask if they are in control? I would like to. Each time someone asks me that, I want to fire the question right back at them.

But for that one moment in the lawyer's office, at least I had remained in control. By not responding to his insensitive comment, I had remained in control of what he would know about me and what judgments he would make about me. What is a temperamental person but a person who lacks control? I would not be that person. But in not being that person, in maintaining that control, I had failed yet again. I had failed myself and everyone else who bears the weight of this label.

PART II

10

Gradually, begrudgingly, but understanding finally that I had no alternative, I joined that legion of people who end up living a life that is very different than the one they had imagined for themselves: women who can't have babies; manic depressives who can't shake the shadows; alcoholics who can't leave the bottle; the millions of people who never knew that just getting through each day could be such a challenge.

The life that I was living was a life that just months before I had not known existed. I could never go back to my old life. I could wish mightily that this had all been a bad dream, that I was going to wake up with a functioning pancreas, but I began to accept that this was not going to happen. I couldn't change the fact that I was dependent upon multiple injections of insulin each day in order to survive. All I could change was how I would deal with it. I would not let it define me. Diabetes would be a part of me, but it would not consume me.

I learned to test my glucose anywhere: on the subway; on a grocery cart, with the meter balanced on top of a grapefruit; at the top of a mountain after a hike; under the conference room table during a meeting. I learned to give myself injections of insulin anywhere, too: in my car when stopped at a red light; in a gondola being transported up a ski slope; in the midst of cooking dinner; doing laundry; and helping Paul's boys with their homework. I learned what all sorts of food and drink did to my glucose level and how to calculate my insulin dosage accordingly. I learned what exercise, sex, stress, and other external factors might do to my glucose level. And I knew that I needed to have my glucose meter, an ample supply of glucose test strips, batteries for the meter, insulin, syringes, glucose pills, and an extra snack with me at all times.

My diabetes began to blend into the fabric of who I was and who I still am. It started to fade into the background. It was always there, and it was never farther away than the back of my mind, but at least there were finally some days when it was not front and center. I guess it was understandable that diabetes took a backseat for a while—I had a wedding to plan.

Paul had asked me to marry him. I accepted tearfully, joyfully, without hesitation. He gave me a stunning sapphire-and-diamond engagement ring. I had never before worn a ring. I spent half of every day with my left arm extended, the palm of my hand facing out, my fingers held up straight, turning my hand slowly left and right, admiring my ring from all angles and in all shades of light. When I rolled my vial of long-acting insulin in my hands each morning to mix it before doing my first shot of the day, I loved the clicking sound that my engagement ring made against the glass vial. That little noise gave me a reason to be happy every morning. It was an audible reminder of the joy of life, with or without diabetes.

A few months after I had started injecting insulin, Paul and I went out to dinner with his boys at a local restaurant. We were getting situated at our table when Ned nudged me, "Amy, look. Look at that lady," he said, gesturing at a woman seated a few tables away.

"Ned, honey, don't point," I responded reflexively. "And why do you want...." My voice trailed off as I realized why Ned had wanted me to look. We all stared. She was using a glucose meter to test her blood sugar. There, in the flesh, just a few feet away, was another person with diabetes. I think, until that moment, we had all labored under the delusion that I was the only one on the planet who had the disease. It sure felt that way most of the time. "I want to talk to her," I said as if in a trance. "Should I go talk to her?" I asked, my gaze still fixed on the woman with the glucose meter.

"Yes. Go. You've got to go talk to her," Paul and the boys answered in a chorus of support.

I rose from our table, my heart beating out of my chest, and approached the woman's table. "I'm so sorry to interrupt," I began. "I couldn't help but notice you testing your blood sugar. And I just wondered if I could talk to you for a few minutes. I was recently diagnosed with diabetes, and..." I hesitated and then continued awkwardly. "I've never talked to another woman who has diabetes."

The woman looked at me kindly. "Please sit down," she said "I'd be happy to talk to you."

"I really don't want to intrude," I stammered.

"Are you taking insulin?" she asked.

"Yes, yes I am."

"Sit," she instructed.

As it turned out, she, too, had Type 1 diabetes. I should have known from her preliminary question about whether I took insulin. I felt like an alien who, after a journey of light-years, across many galaxies, encounters a fellow alien who speaks the same language. She understood highs and lows. She understood short-acting insulin and long-acting insulin. She understood the internal debate that came with every meal in a restaurant, whether to risk the stares of the curious and remain at your table when you squeeze blood from your finger, fill a syringe, and give yourself a shot, or risk the germs and the balancing act of trying to perform these acts in a bathroom stall with no surface but a round toilet paper holder. Talking to her, I realized for the first time that I was not alone. There were others like me.

We shared war stories and statistics: What was your worst low? What's the highest you've ever been? Have you ever lost consciousness?

"What's your A1C?" she asked.

The easy flow of the conversation came to a screeching halt. "My what?"

"Your A1C," she repeated, thinking that I must not have heard her the first time.

"What's an A1C?" I asked. "I don't know what that means."

"You don't know what an A1C is?" she asked "Didn't your doctor tell you what it was when you were diagnosed?"

"No, I don't think so. Or maybe he did, and I missed it. I got a lot of lab results during that initial period. Maybe he told me and I just didn't know what it was."

"Call your doctor tomorrow and ask him what your A1C is," she told me firmly. "You always need to know what your A1C is."

A1C is shorthand for a glycated hemoglobin blood test, which indicates average blood glucose control during the two- to three-month period preceding the test. While a glucose test from a finger prick tells you what your glucose level is at a particular moment in time, the A1C gives you a more thorough picture of overall glucose control during an extended period of time. Depending on its level, an A1C may, among other things, signal that your glucose levels are higher than you think they are between finger pricks, and it may form the basis for adjusting insulin dosages.

Glycated hemoglobin means hemoglobin that has linked up with glucose in the bloodstream. Hemoglobin is found in red blood cells, and its function is to carry oxygen from the lungs to all cells of the body. When glucose levels in the blood are too high, more glucose links up—glycates—with hemoglobin. In a person who doesn't have diabetes, about 5 percent of all hemoglobin is glycated. In a person with diabetes, the A1C percentage can vary widely, from the normal range on up. I have read about, but thankfully have never myself been anywhere close to, A1Cs as high as 15 percent.

The A1C percentage is the single most accurate predictor of whether a person with diabetes will develop complications from the disease. The closer a person's A1C is to the normal range, the less likely it is that he or she will suffer long-term complications from diabetes. An A1C of 7 percent, for example, results in a 50 to 70 percent reduction in the development or progression of retinopathy (eye problems that can lead to blindness), kidney disease, and neuropathy (nerve damage, often in the feet, which can lead to amputation). Most endocrinologists recommend that the goal of insulin therapy should be an A1C of less than 7 percent, and that corrective measures should be taken when the A1C is above that level.

I thanked the kind woman for her information, expressed my most heartfelt appreciation for everything that she had shared with me, and started to excuse myself from her table. Before I did, though, there was just one more thing that I had to ask her.

"Okay, I have just one last question. And it's personal, I hope you don't mind."

"Not at all. Fire away," she said

"Do you have children?" And then, quickly, I asked, "What I mean is, have you ever been pregnant?" Having a brother and a sister who were adopted, I certainly understood there were ways to have children other than as the result of a pregnancy. It was the pregnancy piece, specifically, that I wanted to know about.

"No," she answered, sighing. "No, I haven't ever been pregnant." She glanced across the table at the woman who was her dinner partner and smiled coyly. It occurred to me for the first time since I sat down that perhaps this other woman was her partner for more than dinner. Maybe that was why she had never been pregnant. I hoped that, and not her diabetes, was the reason.

The next day, I called my endocrinologist's office and asked whether an A1C test had been done with my initial lab work. It had not. When I asked my doctor why he had not done this test, he responded that there was no need to do it. He knew the results would be high, because my glucose levels had been so high prior to and during the first few weeks after my diagnosis. I wasn't convinced that was a good enough reason to have not done the test. Even if the result was high, wouldn't we want to know what it was—as a baseline—so that we could monitor improvement based on my treatment? In any event, because I had been on insulin for a few months, he agreed that it was a good time to do the test. I made an appointment and went in the next day. I had my blood drawn and then had three days to wait for the results.

The test assumed a monolithic importance in my mind. I could think of nothing else as I waited those three days. I wanted to hear 7 percent. I wanted to know that all my hard work, the countless finger pricks, and the endless injections of insulin were working.

On the afternoon that my test results were supposed to be ready, I slipped into a phone both in the law school library. I had the proper change for two phone calls: one to the doctor's office and one to Paul, who was expecting my call as soon as I learned the results. I dropped in my first set of coins and punched in the doctor's telephone number. My heart was racing. The doctor was with a patient, but he knew I would be calling in and so he had left my A1C test results with a nurse who picked up the phone.

When she told me my number, I asked her to repeat it so I was sure I had not misheard. She repeated the number. I thanked her, clicked down the receiver just long enough to end the call, and immediately picked it up again and punched in the number to Paul's office. While I was dialing, I started to cry. I couldn't stop the tears

"Amy? Amy, what's wrong? Did you get your results back?"

I tried to catch my breath. "It's working. It's working," I gasped.

"What's working?" Poor Paul, he never knew what I was talking about these days.

"The insulin is working," I sniffed, tears still streaming down my face. "I got a 6.8 percent."

And so I learned another important lesson about living with Type 1 diabetes: hard work pays off. It's tempting some days to just quit trying so hard, to let things slide. The treatment is so relentless, constantly vexing, as the definition of "chronic" had predicted. But to have worked so hard and then to get such positive results made me feel that maybe, somehow, this was all going to work out.

*   *   *

About a year after Paul and I were married, we began to talk seriously about having a baby.

"What does your doctor say?" Paul asked. "About the diabetes, I mean." He didn't need to clarify it—I knew what he meant. "What does she say about having a baby when you have diabetes?"

"She says the sooner, the better. The older I get and the longer I have diabetes, the harder it might be. But for where I am right now, she thinks it should be fine. I'll have to watch my glucose levels more closely."

Even as I said that, I couldn't imagine how I could monitor my glucose levels more frequently than I already did. "My A1C is right where it should be, so she said I can stop taking the pill whenever I want to. And then the second I think I might be pregnant, I have to call her right away. She'll set me up with a specialist who will monitor me throughout the pregnancy."

I knew Paul didn't want to ask the next question. But he had to know. Just as after seeing a purple bruise form and a small lump rise on my thigh several years before, when I had given myself my first shot of insulin, he had asked, "I wonder if they'll all leave a bruise and a bump like that?" The answer then hadn't changed how he felt about me—he just wanted to know what he was dealing with. And so he asked, "What kind of specialist? What kind of problems could there be?"

I could have recited the answer to those questions backward and forward, up and down, coming and going. I knew that pregnancy for a Type 1 diabetic wouldn't be a walk in the park—it's a high-risk endeavor, at best. The mother-to-be risks frequent and unpredictable changes in her glucose levels, and she'll require increasingly greater amounts of insulin, perhaps even having to increase her doses several times in a week. The risks that the mother already faces from having Type 1 diabetes—high blood pressure, heart disease, and kidney failure—will be exacerbated as additional strain is placed on her organs during the pregnancy.

But tell most women these risks, and they probably won't hear them. Here's the question they'll want answered: *What can happen to my baby? What can happen to my baby if my diabetes isn't under control?* A mother would give her heart or her kidneys, would increase her insulin dosage tenfold, would risk her own life, as long as her baby would be healthy.

The first few weeks in the pregnancy of a woman with Type 1 diabetes are crucial. It's during those weeks that the baby's heart, spinal cord, and brain begin to form. Glucose and ketones pass to the developing baby through the placenta, but insulin does not. The baby will be subjected to the mother's high glucose levels but won't have the benefit of the insulin to restore glucose levels to a normal level. Exposure to high glucose levels during this crucial developmental phase can lead to miscarriage or to severe, heartbreaking birth defects.

Later in the pregnancy, after the baby's own pancreas has formed and has begun to produce insulin, the baby may grow very large. If the mother's diabetes is not under control, the baby's blood sugar will be too high. The baby might store the extra glucose as fat and may become big enough to pose risks to the mother and to itself during delivery.

I knew that Paul didn't really want to hear about those risks. We were going to try to have a baby. We had made that decision. He wanted to hear me say that everything was going to be fine. I've always been a fan of the ostrich approach, and at that moment I thought that kicking a little sand over my husband's head might just be the best way to allay his concerns.

"Well, it'll be a high-risk pregnancy. But Dr. Anderson says that as long as I keep my glucose levels under control, I shouldn't have any more problems than a normal—." And then I caught myself. I had accidentally used the word *normal* to refer to someone who doesn't have diabetes. I hated when I did that. I was still normal. I just had diabetes. "I don't mean normal," I corrected myself. "I meant someone who does not have diabetes. Dr. Anderson says that if I keep my blood sugar under control, I shouldn't have any more problems than a woman who doesn't have diabetes."

"I knew what you meant, baby," Paul answered, and he kissed my forehead.

11

One of the best things about my pregnancy was that it didn't take long to happen. Paul and I conceived a baby within weeks. We were about to leave for a spring-break trip to London with Ned, Willie, and a couple of friends when I missed a period. I had also recently begun to experience a few physiological symptoms that made me wonder whether I was pregnant.

We had a new puppy, a belated Christmas gift for Ned and Willie. The puppy was beyond challenging in the house-training department. She broke every rule of nature about an animal not wanting to foul its own den. We were up at least twice each night to clean her crate and to wash poop off her. Yet every day, despite the fact that I was getting very little sleep at night and that when I got home from my law school classes I was always greeted by a poop-smeared pup who again needed cleaning up, I would sit in my classes and think about nothing but the smell of her pink, fuzzy tummy. I stopped going to the library after classes so I could come straight home and take a hit of that puppy-tummy smell. That was clearly not my normal behavior.

Then there was the sleepiness. Certainly part of it could be attributed to the fact that we were up with the puppy several times most nights. But even after those rare nights when I had slept well, I would find myself gazing wistfully at any horizontal surface—a sofa in the law school library, a park bench, a seat on the metro. I struggled to keep away from any place that looked like it would reasonably support a supine human body. I just wanted to lie down, curl up, and sleep whenever and wherever I could.

Last, but certainly not least, particularly from Paul's perspective, I had a nearly insatiable desire to procreate at any given opportunity. I even had the desire when there was not a given opportunity. One cold winter's morning I actually summoned Paul from his car—where he sat in his suit and winter coat, ready to head out to the office—to come back into the house and put me out of my misery. It was this primal urge, more than anything else, that made me think I must be pregnant.

On the day before we departed for London, I decided to buy a home pregnancy test. We would be gone for less than a week, but I wanted to know if I was pregnant before I left the country. I wanted to know if I could drink a pint of lager in a pub or have a glass of wine with dinner. I told myself I would buy the test, but then I would wait for Paul to come home from work before I took it. He should be with me at the moment of truth.

I bought the test. I brought it home and unwrapped it and read all of the instructions. I thought about calling Paul to tell him I had bought the test, but I decided against it. So there was the test kit, sitting on my coffee table. Why was it that I wanted to wait to take the test? I couldn't remember. Now it seemed to make more sense to take the test right away. That way, if I was pregnant, I could call my doctor during business hours and have a quick conversation before I left the country. Yes, I should take the test right away.

I dashed upstairs to the bathroom. Luckily, having diabetes and thus being subject to frequent urination, I could pee almost on command. I never had to wait. And so I dropped my pants, situated myself on the toilet, and peed on the stick. I removed the stick from the stream and started to count the recommended fifteen seconds. I only had to count to three before the result announced itself: a big red plus sign. I got the news that I had longed for and feared in equal measure. I was pregnant.

Pregnant? Oh, my God. Pregnant. Who should I call first—Paul or my doctor? I would call my doctor. I couldn't call Paul and tell him while he was at work. I should wait until he came home. With the same misguided faith in my own powers of self-restraint that made me believe that I could wait until Paul came home before I took the pregnancy test, I told myself that I could wait until he came home to tell him the news. I dialed my doctor's office.

"Hello, yes, I'd like to leave a message for Dr. Anderson to call me, please."

"Okay, what's the message?"

"Well, I just took a pregnancy test, and it came back positive, so I think I'm pregnant. And the doctor said I should call her when I think I'm pregnant."

"Oh, I'll just set up an appointment for you to see her. Sometime in the next month," the receptionist told me.

"No, I need to talk to her right away. I have diabetes. She said I need to talk to her the minute I think I'm pregnant," I responded, trying not to sound desperate but suspecting my tone suggested otherwise.

"Hang on for a second, dear," she said. "I'll see if I can find a nurse."

"Hello," the nurse's voice greeted me after a short period of holding. "You're pregnant, and you have gestational diabetes?" she inquired.

"No. No, I mean, yes, I'm pregnant. But no, I don't have gestational diabetes. I have Type 1 diabetes. I'm insulin-dependent. And I just found out I'm pregnant. The doctor said when it happened that I should call her right away." I was beginning to feel mildly panicked, and I could hear it in my voice. The old unwelcome feeling that I had successfully fought back for so long was rising again.

The nurse responded with an air of gravity that alarmed me, harkening me back to the day of my diagnosis, "Oh, my, I'll have Dr. Anderson call you. I'll have her call you as soon as she can."

"Can you make sure she gets the message today? I'm leaving the country tomorrow, and I'd really like to talk to her today."

"I'll be sure," she answered.

About twenty minutes later my phone rang. It was the doctor. "I understand congratulations are in order." God bless this woman. There wasn't a hint of concern in her voice. There was only happiness. There was only pure joy at the thought of another bun in someone's oven.

"Thank you, thank you," I responded nervously. "Now what do I need to be worried about? About the diabetes I mean. What do I need to do?"

"Just make an appointment to come in tomorrow or the next day, and we'll talk about it then," she answered.

"I can't come in tomorrow or the next day. I'm leaving the country tomorrow. We're going with the boys to London for spring break."

"When are you back?" she asked.

"Next week."

"Well, then come in next week. Make an appointment for the day after you get back. Tell them to fit you in."

"Okay, I will. Is there anything I should be concerned about until then?" I asked.

"Just keep your sugars in tight control. These first few weeks are critical." And then it was as if the doctor could see the petrified expression on my face. "But, Amy, you've got to relax. This is going to be fine. Really, it is. I'll see you next week. Congratulations."

I could not hang up my phone call with the doctor fast enough to call Paul. He answered the phone on the second ring.

"Honey?" I started. "Honey, guess what!"

I didn't leave him time to even start guessing.

"I'm pregnant." I loved hearing myself say these words to him.

"What?" I heard pure joy on his side as well. "Oh, baby, that's wonderful. Just wonderful. I'll try to come home early. I can't wait to tell the boys."

"We can't tell them yet," I responded instantly.

"Why not?"

"It's too early. We need to make sure everything is okay. Let's just go on our trip, and let me see the doctor when we get back, and then we'll tell them when we know everything is okay."

Paul got home a few hours later. Ned and Willie had been home from school for a while and were in the back yard playing while I cooked dinner. Paul came up from behind me and put his arms around my waist.

"There's the little mother-to-be," he said.

"Oh, honey." I turned around to face him, leaned against his chest, and let his arms envelop me. I was weeping silently. He didn't notice until his shirt was nearly soaked through.

"Amy, Amy, what's wrong, baby?" he asked sweetly. "You should be happy. We should be really happy right now."

"I want to be happy. I am happy. But I'm scared," I choked out my answer. "I am just so scared."

12

We left for London the next afternoon. Before we left I picked up a book at one of the airport bookstores: *Midwives: A Novel.* I had chosen it in a rush, based on title only. *How perfect,* I had thought. *A book about midwives. This is just what I want to read on the flight.*

Paul and I had not shared the news of my pregnancy with Ned and Will or with our friends with whom we were traveling. It felt nice and warm to have this little secret with Paul. I just wanted to cozy up to him on the plane, read my book about midwives, and think of our little spawn.

I was not far into the book before I realized that this was not the gentle tale about midwives helping babies into the world that I had imagined. Quite the contrary—it was the horrific yet spellbinding tale of a midwife in rural Vermont who, in order to save a baby, performs an emergency Caesarean section on a woman she believes to have suffered a stroke and died. There is then some question as to whether the mother died of natural causes or whether the midwife killed her when she performed the Caesarean section, and the midwife is charged with murder. The book chronicled the midwife's murder trial. There was so much blood during the Caesarean scene that the pillows on the bed couldn't absorb it all.

All in all, it was not a book I would recommend to a pregnant woman, particularly a suggestible one, like me. Yet I couldn't put the book down. It was an extremely compelling story, and despite the unease that it was causing me, I couldn't wait to read the next turn in the story or the next development in the murder trial. I read all night. I barely slept on the plane.

When we landed I used the bathroom at Heathrow Airport and noticed what I thought was blood on my underpants. *This must be in my imagination*, I told myself. By that point in my life with a chronic health condition, I had garnered at least enough self-awareness to know that I'm more than susceptible to the power of suggestion. The bloody, gory scene from the novel must have captured my imagination so fully that I actually thought I was bleeding. *What a nut I am. It's going to be a long nine months if I think something's wrong every time I use the bathroom.* I convinced myself that it was nothing and left the airport bathroom to rejoin my family.

Thinking it would be better to keep everyone awake and active in order to get ourselves acclimated to London time, we decided to do a little sightseeing straight away rather than going to sleep, which is what our bodies were begging us to do. Our first stop was Madame Tussauds wax museum, culminating with a nauseating ride through the Chamber of Horrors, which offered a bloody tribute to murderers from the dawn of time. There was even an entire section devoted to infamous serial killers. The street where Jack the Ripper once roamed through the East End of London was reproduced in terrifyingly realistic detail, right down to a heavy fog that enveloped the observer. We were all transported through the gore-fest in a vehicle that looked, in roughly equal parts, like a train in a horror movie and a kiddie roller coaster in a traveling carnival.

However, the roller-coaster aspect of it may be a fiction that my memory has created based on my perception of the ride. I was sitting next to one of the boys, though I don't remember which one. And I thought I was going to die. Or at the very least, I thought I was going to vomit. I desperately did not want to vomit on whichever of the boys was sitting next to me, and I certainly didn't want to vomit on the back of the stranger who was sitting in front of me. Yet with each twist and then again with each turn, and certainly again with each bloodstained killer's figure that popped out to startle us, my stomach rose closer to my throat. I needed to stop moving. I needed to get off the damned ride. I contemplated stepping out of the car when it was at a slow point. What would happen to me then? The ride would go on, Ned or Willie, whoever I was next to, would panic, and I would be left alone in the Chamber of Horrors. Would the already dim light be extinguished altogether, and would I then have to feel my way out along the track, pausing periodically to vomit along my way?

Before I could think my way out of that desperate situation, we exited the Chamber of Horrors, and the ride lurched to a stop. I stood up too quickly, ready to bolt, but I was dizzy and nearly lost my balance. I put my hand out to steady myself on the wall. I was green. Not figuratively green, but actually green. Paul rushed to my side. "Are you okay?" he asked.

"That ride just didn't sit well with me," I said, trying to shrug it off and right myself. I didn't want our friends to know I was suffering from a wicked bout of morning sickness, compounded by an overactive imagination that was replaying the scene of the botched Caesarean. All aspects of the Chamber of Horrors had exacted their toll on me.

"Maybe we should go take a rest," our friends offered. "The boys look tired, too. I think some downtime would do us all some good."

I looked over at Ned and Willie, who were glassy-eyed. They were right. I didn't need to hear that suggestion twice. "Great idea," I said. "Let's go to the hotel."

Once there, Paul and I fell immediately into our bed, and Ned and Will hopped into theirs. We were all asleep within minutes. We slept soundly, the four of us, in our one little hotel room, in our two double beds, for some time.

I was the first to wake up. I lay still for several minutes, listening to the peaceful sounds of Paul and the boys breathing. I loved listening to them sleep. It was so rare for the four of us to be so quiet, so still, and so together in one space. I treasured those rare moments. Then, rolling over to cuddle up to Paul, I felt a sensation that is not foreign to any menstruating woman. I felt a warm bulb of blood slide out of my body. I realized that that sensation is what had awakened me. I froze mid-roll. *That felt very real*, I thought to myself. *That felt like a figment of something, but not of my imagination.*

Slowly, as quietly as I could, I eased myself out of bed and tip-toed across the room to the one bathroom that we all shared. I closed the door, locked it, and pulled my pants down. I was greeted by what I feared most: blood. Not overactive-imagination blood, not may-be-you-are-making-this-up blood, but real blood. Thick, red blood. Period blood. I pulled my pants back up, unlocked the door, and hurried back into bed with Paul. I woke him up, in a loud whisper, trying not to wake the boys and told him.

"What should we do?" he asked. "Do you think we should find a doctor for you?"

I didn't know what we should do any more than Paul did. "No, I don't think so," I answered. "I'm not sure what the point of seeing a doctor would be. I'm only about six weeks pregnant. So maybe I'm miscarrying. If I am, I don't think there's anything a doctor can do at this stage. If I'm not, and everything is fine, then it doesn't matter either way."

I said all of that logically, as if the problem were an exercise in deductive reasoning. I felt anything but logical, however, as I clamped my legs together tightly, shut my eyes, and silently prayed that our precious fertilized egg was still inside me. I thought about several high glucose levels, well into the high 200s, that I had endured over the past few weeks, before I knew I was pregnant. Would those have been enough to throw off the pregnancy? I had no idea.

I passed the rest of our London vacation in a restless state. The bleeding continued, sometimes faintly, but at other times more heavily. I was exhausted with worry. Our traveling companions knew there was something wrong, but they didn't know what. They were concerned that my diabetes had taken a turn for the worse. They noticed that I was more careful than usual about what I ate, that I declined lager at pubs, and that I tested my glucose levels more often than usual. They noticed that I was tired, more so than normal jet lag would explain, and often distracted. They noticed me and Paul talking in hushed tones after I used the bathroom, when I was reporting back to him about my condition.

A few days into the bleeding, I decided to buy a pregnancy test. I didn't know whether or not the test would be foolproof; I supposed it was possible for it to show a false positive for some period of time during or after a miscarriage. But I did know it would make me feel better. That afternoon, after we had lunch (or rather, after the others had lunch and I had picked and hemmed and hawed as I tried to guess what fish and chips would do to my glucose level), we went back to the hotel to let the boys have a little downtime. While Paul and the boys rested, I stole away to the chemist across the street and bought a pregnancy test.

I returned to our hotel room and went into the small bathroom with my bag from the chemist. I tried to muffle the crackle of the paper as I opened the bag and to blunt the crinkle of the plastic as I unwrapped the test kit. I peed on the stick, and for the second time in just one week felt grateful for my ever-present ability to urinate. I closed my eyes, counted, and waited. When I got to ten, I opened my eyes and looked down at the stick. I saw a plus sign. The test was positive. It was telling me I was still pregnant.

I will never tire of shedding tears of joy. They are the best kind of tears there are, and recently I had cried more than my share: tears for my good A1C percentage; tears for my marriage proposal; tears for my first positive pregnancy test. And there I was, crying again, for my second positive pregnancy test.

13

I saw Dr. Anderson the day after we returned from London. She did a pregnancy test and confirmed that I was indeed still pregnant. "But why all the bleeding?" I asked.

"Well, it could be any number of things. My guess would be that it's just implantation bleeding," she answered.

"What's that?" I asked.

"Implantation is when the fertilized egg implants, or attaches, to the uterus. It can cause bleeding in some women when the lining of the uterus is disturbed. If the egg isn't able to implant on the first try, it may move to another spot, and then the first spot, where it didn't attach, may bleed for a while."

"How do we know if that's the cause?"

"In your case, I'd like to do an ultrasound, just to get a better look."

"Okay," I said. And then I asked, "Umm, doctor, is this because of my diabetes?" This is a question I always have to ask. No matter what the symptom. If I have a headache: Is this because of my diabetes? If I am very tired: Is this because of my diabetes? If I am moody: my diabetes? Now that the embryo that was my little baby was having a hard time finding a place to implant itself—was that because of my diabetes? I think what I was trying to understand was—Do I just have bad luck? Or do I have really, really bad luck—like born-under-a-bad-sign bad luck?

The doctor looked at me patiently, sympathetically. "It probably has nothing to do with your diabetes. This happens to lots of women. It's very common. Now, before you leave today, just tell the person at the front desk that you need to schedule an ultrasound, and she'll give you the referral and the contact information to set up the appointment." Then the doctor dug around in the pocket of her lab coat for a prescription pad, wrote down the name and phone number of another doctor, and handed the paper to me. "And this is the perinatologist whom I want you to call. He's terrific. You'll really like him."

"I don't get it. What does he do? What's a perinatologist? I want you to be my doctor." I said the last bit teasingly, but I meant it. I did not want to go through all of this with a new doctor.

"Not to worry. I'll still be your doctor. I'll see you through your pregnancy, and I will deliver your baby. Dr. Landini, the perinatologist, is a high-risk specialist. His job is to help you manage your diabetes throughout your pregnancy. You'll probably talk to him lots more often than you talk to me. Depending on how things go, you may even talk to him every day."

"When should I call him?" I asked.

"Call him today," the doctor answered "He'll want to start getting your glucose levels right away."

After the doctor's assistant took a blood sample to run some routine screening tests, I stopped by the front desk to schedule my next appointment and to pick up the ultrasound information. The young lady at the front desk gave me a little bag of informational brochures, coupons, and the like for the mother-to-be. "Congratulations," she said cheerily as she handed me the bag full of goodies.

"Thanks very much," I responded, somewhat halfheartedly as I took the bag. My excitement at being pregnant was being weighed down by Dr. Anderson's instructions to call the perinatologist right away and by her comment that I would likely be talking to him very often. It made me concerned that maybe this pregnancy was riskier than anyone was letting on. What I didn't realize then but what became apparent to me over the course of my pregnancy was that I should have been comforted, not alarmed, by the fact that I would have such frequent interactions with a high-risk specialist. That didn't mean I was worse off than I imagined. It meant that I was going to get the best medical care available to manage my glucose levels for the next thirty weeks or so. It meant that my baby and I just might get through the pregnancy without any complications.

I called Dr. Landini's office as soon as I got home. I spoke with his assistant, and it was instantly apparent that she was very experienced in dealing with women with Type 1 diabetes. It was always a welcome relief to find someone who talks the talk of the insulin-dependent diabetic. She knew all about the different kinds of insulin that I was taking, and she understood what different glucose levels meant. She wasn't alarmed or confused by anything I said. She asked me how much and what type of insulin I was taking, and at what times of day I took it. At that time I was giving myself one injection of long-acting insulin before breakfast each morning and injections of short-acting insulin before lunch and dinner.

She asked me what my glucose levels had been like lately. I read to her from my logbook my glucose levels for the prior day. I routinely recorded my glucose levels upon waking, before each meal, and at bedtime. I had also performed and recorded four to five other glucose tests throughout the day as circumstances required. I read my scores proudly; they all sounded great to me.

"Okay, we're going to need to work on those," she said

"Work on those?" I asked, somewhat defensively. "I thought they looked pretty good. I mean, for me, anyway, those are pretty good numbers."

"Maybe before you were pregnant, but now we want you below 100 before every meal," she responded efficiently.

Below 100? The words reverberated in my head. How could I keep my glucose level below 100? That sounded awfully close to 90, and 90 sounded awfully close to 80, and 80 was way too close to 70. And we all know what 70 means.

"And what are your postprandials?" she asked.

"My what?" I responded. I had no idea what she was talking about. Over the years that I have lived with this disease, I have learned not to be surprised by what I do not know. But back then, in the early years, I believed I could master it simply by learning everything that there was to know. So I was caught off guard whenever I heard a term that was new to me. If I didn't know what postprandial meant, what else did I not know? Any ignorance could affect not only me but also my baby, and that made learning suddenly much more important.

"Your postprandials—your glucose levels after meals. What are your numbers like after meals?"

"I don't know," I said slowly, the wheels in my head starting to turn. "I don't usually check after meals." I knew where she was going. I was going to need to start checking after meals. That would add three more glucose tests to the eight or so that I was already doing every day.

"We're going to need you to check your glucose level one hour after every meal. And we're going to want see 130 or lower at that one-hour mark," she told me matter-of-factly.

I remembered the conversation with my doctor a few months earlier, when I told her that Paul and I were ready to try to have a baby. She had said I would need to keep my glucose levels in very tight control. Before I was pregnant, tight control meant a glucose level under 120 before meals and under 180 two hours after a meal. Those numbers were aggressive for me, but often I achieved them. My good A1C result was proof that my glucose levels were staying in a normal range much of the time. The numbers that this assistant was telling me sounded unrealistic, unattainable. I could not imagine how I would achieve the level of control she described.

Gathering my thoughts, trying to absorb what she was telling me, I asked what the next steps were.

"I'll schedule you for an appointment to come in and see the doctor later this week. For now, just keep writing down your glucose levels. And don't forget to check an hour after every meal. Call us if you're high after meals. Or if you seem to be high at other times."

"What do you mean by 'high?'" I asked. As an insulin-dependent diabetic, you always have to ask this question. High is not just what the pamphlets tell you it is. High is all relative. One hundred forty might be high for someone who is trying to keep very tight control, 180 might be high for someone who is focusing on getting her A1C down, and 220 might be high but bearable for someone who is afraid of being low. I didn't know what high meant for a pregnant woman.

"Above 150," she answered. "So if we don't hear from you before, we'll see you at your appointment the day after tomorrow."

I hung up the phone. Above 150 was high? The words bounced around in my head. My glucose level was above 150 many hours of each day. It was not unusual for me to have a glucose level over 200 after meals.

Staying below 150 would mean exercising a level of restraint and control beyond the already-vigilant practices that I had grown accustomed to. It would mean measuring out my food servings so I would be sure I was eating a correct portion size for purposes of calculating my insulin dosage. It would mean that mistakes in insulin dosage—which are easy to make when the hash marks that demark a unit of insulin on a syringe are about one millimeter apart—would take on a new significance. It would mean no popping a handful of grapes or popcorn into my mouth casually, without counting the pieces out and injecting a tiny dose of insulin to cover them. It would mean that a low was around every corner and that there was no buffering against it—no overeating or under-dosing so that I could have the temporary security of not worrying about a low. It would mean doubling up on my finger-pricking when I was above 150, so I would know whether my glucose level was staying too high or starting to fall.

It would mean having a great deal of faith in my medical team, who would increase my insulin dosage to levels that prior to my pregnancy would have landed me in the emergency room or worse.

Below 150. She had said I had to keep my glucose level below 150. Those old feelings of confusion and panic, my constant companions in the weeks and months following my diagnosis, those two that I had not missed in the least since they had left me—they were back with a vengeance.

14

Technological advances in the treatment of diabetes over the course of the past century have been no less dramatic than the transition from the hi-fidelity stereo to the iPod. If I had been a person with Type 1 diabetes in the early 1900s, I probably wouldn't have lived long enough to write this book. I might have been put on a starvation diet, which could have prolonged my life for a few years. A starvation diet is just what the name implies: a diet that severely restricts caloric intake—enough to keep the glucose level in check for a period of time but ultimately not enough to sustain life for more than several years.

If I had been born in the 1920s, I might have been one of the first fortunate few to be treated with insulin. I would have used glass syringes with large-bore needles to inject it, and I would have had to boil my needles to sterilize them. I would have used a pumice stone to file them down after each use. I would have used this tool, which is better suited for softening a callous on the foot, to try to hone to a fine point the needle that I would need to use again in just a few short hours to inject the insulin that would keep me alive. I would have had to do this as many times a day as I had to give myself injections.

I wouldn't have been able to prick my finger and see the accurate glucose level that I see today on my glucose meter. Rather, I would have tested my urine for sugar levels. Each day I would have saved a specimen of my urine in a cup and then dipped a test strip into it. Based on the color that the strip turned, I would have tried to estimate what my glucose level was. The level would not have been a real-time measure; it would have been a measure from some indeterminate number of hours before, depending on how long the urine had been stored in my bladder. If my glucose level were not above 180, the urine test would not show my glucose level as high. If my glucose level were too low, it would not register at all. If I had taken a vitamin or some other medication that changed the color of my urine, the test result may have been unreliable altogether.

But I would have tested my urine. I would have starved myself, boiled my syringes, filed my needles, and endured the barbaric injections. I would have done all of those things religiously. I would have hoped and prayed that in doing so, I would live longer than the thirteen years that the first person who ever injected insulin to treat Type 1 diabetes had survived.

It's a difficult thing for a woman whose pancreas produces no insulin to be told that she has to keep her post-meal glucose level below 150. But thanks to the development of a fast-acting insulin around that time, I might be able to do just that. The new insulin was assimilated rapidly, just ten to thirty minutes after injection, then peaked and was out of the system within about two hours. This enabled people with diabetes to cut out a lot of the guesswork involved with trying to time meals around longer-acting insulin that peaked thirty to sixty minutes after injection and then remained active in the body for several more hours.

Gone also were the days when people with diabetes had to know what they were going to eat well in advance of the meal so they could gauge their insulin dosage accordingly. The new type of insulin could be injected essentially right before a meal. Once you saw what you were going to be eating, you could approximate the right dosage and cover that meal. If you were too high after the meal, you could bump your glucose level down pretty quickly with a corrective injection after you finished eating.

I began taking that new insulin right after my first appointment with the perinatologist. I showed up for my appointment a few days after my initial telephone conversation with his nurse, armed with the log of all of my pre-meal, post-meal, and all-times-in-between glucose levels for the days since I had spoken with her. My glucose levels had been good: A few were close to being too high, a few were close to being too low, but all in all, I was happy with them. I was, nevertheless, feeling nervous to meet another doctor who would analyze how I was controlling my diabetes.

I sat in the waiting room and waited for my name to be called. I had to wait longer than I would have liked, but I told myself that it was a good thing. That must mean the perinatologist spends a lot of time with each patient. Finally the receptionist announced, "Mrs. Ryan? Dr. Landini will see you now." I rose and walked back to the examination room.

The first thing I noticed about Dr. Landini was that he was quite easy on the eyes. I knew instantly that I would always look forward to coming to see him because I could, well, see him. When he introduced himself to me, I learned that he was also easy on the ears. He had an Italian accent and a very gentle voice. Perhaps this high-risk pregnancy business was not going to be as dreadful as I had imagined. I could already see at least one upside.

The doctor examined my medical history thoroughly. He explained the risks for a pregnant woman with Type 1 diabetes, which I already knew, along with the risks for my developing baby, some of which frightened the hell out of me. Then he performed a sonogram and confirmed, as my obstetrician had suspected, that my bleeding was implantation bleeding. He showed me on the computer screen, as he rolled the sonogram sensor over my belly, the spot in my uterus where the baby had tried unsuccessfully to implant. My little trooper had moved on and found a more secure spot in another part of my uterus.

"There's your baby," the doctor said, holding the sensor firmly against my belly. Looking at the computer screen, I was surprised to see that my baby did not look like a tadpole, which for some reason is what I expected. It also did not look quite like a baby. But it did look like a little living thing. It definitely looked like a living creature. It had been hard to believe at times that there was a little somebody alive inside of me, what with the bleeding and the lack of feeling any movement. However, when I saw the little creature on the sonogram screen, its heart pumping away, any doubts I might have felt vanished immediately. There was our baby. That was the little creature whose glucose level I had to keep normal for about thirty more weeks.

After finishing the sonogram the doctor handed me a tissue to wipe the gel off of my belly, and then waited for me to readjust my clothes before turning on the light in the room. After I was situated and the lights were back on, the doctor went over my glucose levels with me. He asked me what types of insulin I was taking. He explained there was a new fast-acting insulin that could be injected shortly before each meal. He wanted me to start using it. These shots would be in addition to the injection of longer-acting insulin that I gave myself upon waking each morning.

"Start on that, and then call in two days with your pre- and postprandial glucose levels," he told me. "And I'm going to want you to call in every Monday, Wednesday, and Friday with your glucose levels. We'll also schedule more frequent lab work to get your A1Cs, and we will schedule more sonograms as the baby develops," he continued.

I understood the A1Cs, but I was not sure about the sonograms. "Why more sonograms?" I asked.

"We'll want to check the spine, measure the limbs, and measure the head regularly to make sure the baby is developing on course," he answered. He wasn't specific, but the scary possibilities that accompanied scientific measurement made my stomach wrench. I knew that babies born to women who have Type 1 diabetes were more prone to birth defects than babies whose mothers did not have diabetes. For me, anyway, the statistical incidence of these birth defects was of little comfort: The fact that they might happen at all, however remote the chances, was all I needed to know. If it could happen to one baby, it could happen to mine.

The specific baby body parts that he had mentioned brought home the reality of what could happen, of what could go wrong.

He would check the spine for signs of spina bifida or other spinal defects. He would measure the limbs for signs that one or more of the baby's arms or legs would be malformed. He would measure the head for any indication that the baby was getting too large and may be difficult to deliver.

Miscarriages and stillbirths also occur more frequently in pregnancies where mothers have Type 1 diabetes, and the doctor reminded me of this fact. My thoughts leapt to the unsettling conclusion that a good report at my appointment one week would not guarantee that there would still be a baby to check at the next appointment. The cold, hard truth was that a full nine months of constant vigilance would not necessarily guarantee a live baby at the end. In that moment, it became clear that I was going to have a lot more to wrestle with than my glucose levels during my pregnancy.

15

I started on the new insulin the day after my first appointment with Dr. Landini. I gave myself insulin injections faithfully four or five times a day and tested my glucose levels compulsively. I ate much the same thing, at the same time, at every meal, from one day to the next: an egg, an English muffin, and eight ounces of skim milk for breakfast; a turkey sandwich, an apple, and eight ounces of skim milk for lunch; and for dinner, a serving of protein, pasta or rice, and a vegetable—if I had kept up with the grocery shopping and had anything fresh in the refrigerator. It was easier to maintain a normal glucose level, to stay below 150, without variations in my diet. It wasn't the time to try new foods or to eat a late breakfast or to skip lunch. My diet had to be managed with a monotonous degree of precision.

I called Dr. Landini's office every Monday, Wednesday, and Friday. I would talk to a nurse, give her my glucose levels, and then get a call back with any adjustments in my insulin doses. The adjustments were more frequent than I would have liked. I was always leery of taking a larger dose of insulin, because I was so afraid of the low that might follow. But I followed the doctor's instructions, and the lows were few and far between.

One low that I do recall was on the day of my graduation from law school. As a matter of fact, it was literally during my graduation ceremony, when my law school class section was being awarded diplomas. The diplomas were awarded in alphabetical order. The announcer was up to the Ds. I was an R, because by that time I was using my married name, Ryan. (Thank goodness I was not still an F for Fitzgerald, or I may have missed receiving my diploma altogether.) I began to feel the familiar, dreaded sense of a pressing vacancy descending upon me. A heavy cloud of confusion was settling over the proceedings.

Maybe it's the heat, I told myself. It was Memorial Day weekend (three years, to the weekend, after my diagnosis) in Washington, D.C. It must have been 95 degrees in the shade, and I was not in the shade. I was baking with the rest of my class on a concrete patio. I was four months pregnant. I had on a maternity dress—my first, which I was not quite physically ready for, but I had just outgrown my non-maternity clothes—and that added yards of fabric beneath my black graduation gown. So I tried to convince myself that maybe I was just hot. Surely the heat was why I was sweating. Maybe I wasn't really low.

So began the mental game that accompanies my lows. Am I low, or am I just overheated? Should I do a glucose test, or should I not? In most settings, I would always err on the side of caution and do a glucose test. But there, in my graduation gown, sitting among my classmates, the last thing I wanted to do was to pull out my glucose meter, prick my finger, and perhaps draw attention to myself. I had carried my glucose meter with me, tucked away under the large cuff of the sleeve of my graduation gown.

I waited until the roll caller got to the Gs, and I wasn't feeling any better. My thoughts weren't connecting. I pulled out my glucose meter as surreptitiously as possible, pricked my finger, and waited for the result. I heard the beep, which I had tried to muffle under my robe, and looked down at the screen: 63.

Damn it. That was all I could think. *Damn it. Damn it. It's my graduation from law school, I'm minutes away from being awarded my diploma, and I'm low. Damn it. I am low at my law school graduation. Goddamn it.*

For one of the very few times in my lifetime with diabetes, I did not have any glucose pills with me. Although I had carried my glucose meter with me, I had not wanted the additional burden of a bottle of glucose pills, because that would have meant carrying a purse. No woman carries a purse when she processes in her cap and gown. Even people with diabetes have a modicum of dignity and fashion sense.

I didn't think that I could make it from the Gs to the Rs without getting some glucose in me. My name could be ten to fifteen minutes off, and by that time I might not know where I was or why my name was being called. I didn't want to risk it. I stood up and worked my way past my classmates and out of the row of seats. I found Paul, the boys, and my family sitting nearby.

"What are you doing?" Paul asked in a loud whisper, alarmed.

"I'm low," I said urgently.

"Where are your pills?" Paul asked.

"I don't have any. Give me some money—I'll go get a soda." I had spied a cafeteria or snack bar near the area where my class section was seated.

"Let me get it," Paul said "You're going to miss your diploma."

"No, I'll get it," I insisted. I can't say whether my insistence was obstinacy brought on by my low, or whether I wanted to prove that I could still take care of myself. I think it was the latter. I think I needed to show myself that I could feel my low, treat it, and get back in time to collect my diploma. I needed to be able to take care of myself. I needed my diabetes not to interfere with that day, and I needed to be the one who prevented it from interfering.

Paul handed me two one-dollar bills and some change. "Hurry," he said, and I rushed to the snack bar. I bought a Sprite, opened it even before I had paid, and drank half of it before leaving the store. I made my way back among my classmates and took my seat, sipping on the second half of my Sprite as the announcer moved closer to the Rs. When she got to the Os, I pricked my finger again. To heck with modesty. I wanted to make sure I was stable when my name was called. I looked down at the flashing hourglass on the screen of my glucose meter, awaiting the beep, which finally came: 108. I had recovered. I was going to be okay.

The roll call proceeded. Moments later I heard my name: "Amy Fitzgerald Ryan, cum laude." I walked forward amid the polite applause from the general audience, but what I heard was the whooping of Paul, the boys, and my family. I shook the hand of the presenter and received my diploma.

In the photographs from my graduation, I have a bottle of Sprite in my hand. I also have an unmistakable look of pride.

*   *   *

The next few months of my pregnancy were uneventful. In the life of a pregnant woman, and particularly in the life of a pregnant woman who has Type 1 diabetes, uneventful is good. I spent the first half of the summer studying for the bar exam. Compared to my schedule during the school year, when I had been in law school and Ned and Willie were in school and I was running them around to various after-school activities, studying for the bar exam was a breeze. I went to a review class every morning for a few hours, and then came home and had the afternoons to myself. For the first time in years, I had a few hours to relax every day. And relax I did.

I took the bar exam for the Commonwealth of Virginia in July, following my graduation from law school. Virginia is one of the few jurisdictions that requires people who sit for the bar exam to dress as if they were appearing in court. That is, coat and ties for the gentlemen, dresses or suits for the ladies. I splurged and bought a high-end maternity suit with a jacket, reasoning that I could wear it again when I started work a few months later.

When I received my registration materials for the bar exam, I noticed a statement directed to test takers who had special needs or would require special accommodations. I did not like to think of myself as someone who had a disability. Surely, and indeed legally, my diabetes was a disability. I had a physical impairment that substantially limits a major life activity. My pancreas doesn't produce insulin. I cannot survive without injections of insulin. But I have never wanted to admit that I might need special accommodations.

A few days before the bar exam, I started getting nervous. The exam would take two full days. I would be seated in a proctored testing room for eight hours per day on two consecutive days. Depending on the seating arrangements, I might not be comfortable doing a glucose test at my seat. Would I be allowed to take my glucose meter into the bathroom? What if I decided to do a glucose test at my seat after all, and the beep from my meter disturbed another test taker? What if my glucose level fell too low during the test and I was not able to concentrate? What if I needed time to recover? What if...? What if...?

I asked Paul what he thought I should do. Should I arrange for special accommodations? "You'll be fine, babe, you'll be fine," was his answer. Perhaps I had proven myself too capable of handling my diabetes. He gave me no special attention whatsoever.

In the end, I did not ask for special accommodations. I took breaks when I needed to and checked my glucose levels when I needed to in the privacy of a stall in the ladies' room. There was never a question as to the little black pouch that I carried with me. My glucose level was fine for the two days of the exam. I didn't have any lows or any worrisome highs.

During one of my trips to the ladies' room, another woman, a fellow test taker, noticed that I was pregnant. I was into my fifth month by then, and in my maternity suit, there was really no mistaking it. "Oh my God, you're *pregnant?*" she said to me. It was unusual to see a pregnant woman sitting for the bar exam.

"Yep, I am," I responded. What else could I say?

"Oh my God," she said again, as if the first time she said this she had not made her point. "I feel so sorry for you."

I didn't know what to make of her comment. I thought she must mean that she felt sorry for me having to wear a suit and sit in a testing room for eight hours when I was pregnant. But her comment hadn't really come out that way. I was not sure how to respond. She stood facing me.

"Oh, don't," I stammered. "Don't feel sorry for me. We're all in the same boat," I said congenially and then continued on my way.

Feel sorry for me? I wondered as I walked away. I pondered this concept long after our encounter had ended. She didn't know the half of it. But even if she had, why should anyone feel sorry for me? I was pregnant, I had a husband who adored me, and I had two healthy stepsons. I was the luckiest person on Earth. I should be envied, not pitied, shouldn't I?

16

After the bar exam was over, I had the entire month of August free. I wasn't scheduled to start work at my new job until after Labor Day. By that time my insulin dosages had increased significantly. I had been calling Dr. Landini's office and reporting my glucose levels three times a week, as instructed. Before I was pregnant, I had been injecting myself with two to three units of short-acting insulin before lunch and before dinner. By August, I was injecting myself with nearly fifteen units of short-acting insulin before breakfast, before lunch, and before dinner. Those three injections were in addition to the injection of long-acting insulin that I gave myself when I woke up every morning.

At the start of my pregnancy I would never have believed anyone who told me that my insulin doses would have increased sevenfold. Honestly, I would have thought that fifteen units of insulin before a meal could have killed me. But because my insulin dosages were increased gradually over a number of months and always under the careful monitoring of the high-risk specialist and his staff, I was managing successfully what otherwise wouldn't have been a manageable pregnancy.

I don't recall for certain how frequently I saw Dr. Landini in his office. I'm sure that, in my memory, the visits were more frequent than they were in reality. Those appointments were in addition to my appointments with Dr. Anderson, my obstetrician. I still saw my obstetrician for the typical pregnancy exams. I saw the high-risk specialist for something that, in my estimation, was far more crucial.

Each time I saw him, he did a thorough, slow, detailed sonogram, measuring each joint-to-joint segment in my baby's body. I would lie on the examining table, watching the sonogram screen as he marked off measurements that I could see on the screen but which to me were indecipherable. He measured the baby's head from many different perspectives: the circumference of the head around the forehead; the distance from one side to the other on the widest part of the baby's head; the length of the baby's head from crown to chin. He measured the baby's spine. He measured the length of the baby's shoulder to elbow, and elbow to wrist, first measuring one little arm and then the other. He measured the length of the baby's hip to knee, and knee to ankle, first measuring one little leg and then the other.

Dr. Landini had a poker face. He didn't betray anything, and I hardly breathed while he took those measurements. At the end of each intensive session he told me, "Your baby looks fine, Amy. Your baby looks just fine." Each time I heard this, I could scarcely keep my emotions in check long enough to make it to my car in the parking lot before I burst into tears. *We are really going to do it, this baby and I. We are really going to make it,* I would think.

Paul went with me to one of my later sonograms. He had not been to a lot of the earlier ones because there were just too many, and there wasn't that much to see. I'm not one of those women who believed that "we" were pregnant. Paul was not pregnant. Paul's ankles weren't swelling; his hormones weren't raging; he wasn't gaining weight. Only I was pregnant. The doctor's appointments were mine. For the most part, and given the number of medical appointments that I had, it was easier for me to deal individually with the doctors than to try to involve Paul in all of my appointments. But by September, when I was in my third and final trimester, it seemed to make sense for Paul to get another look at the baby and to see how far we had come.

Having already fathered two boys, Paul was no stranger to sonogram images. But it had been many years, more than eight, since he had seen one. And he couldn't recall ever having seen one so far along in the gestational process. Paul was shocked to find, when he saw the baby on the screen, that what he saw was... a baby. It was real. It was defined. It looked as if it could have grabbed a rattle and shaken it around if someone would just hand it one. Paul's amazement was not lost on Dr. Landini.

"Would you like to know the sex of your baby?" the doctor asked.

"Yes," Paul said.

"No," I said.

We had talked about this for the past six months, and we had agreed that we did not want to know the sex of the baby. We wanted to be surprised. I envisioned a traditional delivery. Again, here, ignorance was bliss—I don't know whether there really is such a thing as a traditional delivery. I imagined my baby being delivered, the doctor joyfully announcing, "It's a boy" or "It's a girl," and then delivering a slap on the bottom to set the baby wailing. During this time Paul and I would be gazing at each other lovingly, me looking tired but more alive and beautiful than ever, while we waited for the staff to hand us our cleaned-up and quieted baby, who would begin suckling, effortlessly, right away. Imagination and hope are very significant elements of childbearing.

So I was surprised to hear Paul say that he wanted to know the baby's sex.

"I thought you didn't want to know," I reminded him.

"I didn't," he said. "But look at it.... No, I can't even call it 'it' anymore. That's a real baby. I need to know if it's a girl or a boy. I need to call it 'he' or 'she.'"

The doctor looked at me. I looked at Paul. "Are you sure?" I asked.

"Yes," he answered. Paul is always sure.

"Okay, you can tell us," I told the doctor. What he told us would be accurate. For reasons unrelated to my diabetes, I had had an amniocentesis earlier in my pregnancy. The results of this test, not just the doctor's best impression based on my sonogram, would confirm the sex indisputably.

Dr. Landini paused, allowing us to consider our decision and allowing the drama to build for just a few moments. "You're having a girl," he said. "Your baby is a little girl."

17

In September, a few months after my graduation from law school and a few months shy of my due date, I started work as an associate at a law firm in Washington, D.C.—not the same law firm that employed the person who had made the reference to "temperamental diabetics" the year before. It is highly unusual for a woman to show up for her first day of work at a law firm seven months pregnant. When a woman finishes law school, passes the bar exam, and then starts a job at a world-renowned firm, people do not usually say, "That's great. You should have a baby now. As a matter of fact, you should be noticeably pregnant when you show up for your first day of work."

In major metropolitan law firms, job offers to law students typically are made at the end of the summer after a law student's second year of law school. If the student performs well for a law firm during that summer, the firm more often than not will extend an offer of employment to commence during the fall of the year that the student graduates. Under this regime, job offers are given and accepted twelve to eighteen months before the anticipated start date.

Most law students work as summer associates at law firms following their second year of law school. I was fortunate enough to work as a summer associate following my first year as well. I had been in that position for only a matter of weeks when I began to suspect that I had made a grievous error in judgment by starting law school at the age of thirty, when I already had two stepchildren. I was also in my prime childbearing years, and I found myself with a serious health condition that made it imperative I have a child earlier rather than later.

I also found myself in a profession that, especially in 1990, was not exactly welcoming to pregnant women—or, for that matter, to women who already had children and wished to see them awake at some point before they went off to college. To top it off, I found myself during that summer working at a law firm at which I do not recall anyone mentioning their family or leaving work at a reasonable hour to see their kids—least of all women, who had to prove that they were committed above all else to their profession and that they would not be derailed by the demands of motherhood.

I could express my despair only to Paul. Should I cut my losses, give up on this law school lark, and try to do something else that might leave me time to have a family life? Paul, a lawyer himself, knew how hard I had worked. He knew how well I had done. He didn't want me to throw in the towel. Paul was more attuned than I to law firms in Washington, D.C., and he told me about one that was known as being a family-friendly firm in an era before family friendly became a buzz phrase. This firm was supposedly a great place for women, a great place for parents—it even had a daycare center on site in its main office.

"Why don't you send them a résumé?" he said "It's worth a shot. See if you can work there next summer."

I have had my share of bad luck in my life—perhaps more than my share. At the same time, I have not wanted for lucky breaks, either. I sent my résumé, the firm called me in for an interview, and I ended up working there the following summer. My experience there could not have been more different than my experience a summer earlier.

Lawyers at my new law firm had families, and they talked about those families. Men and women alike celebrated their children and arranged their schedules in a way that allowed them to be parents and lawyers. The management took a novel and innovative approach to integrating firm life with family life, and the difference in the day-to-day atmosphere there was palpable.

During that summer, I had lunch with a female attorney who had worked at the firm for a few years. She told me she had been pregnant with her first child when she started work. I nearly choked on my pad thai. "What?" I asked, certain that I had misheard her. "You were pregnant when you started?" I was incredulous. Most women would've said you shouldn't have a baby during your first five years of practice, not to mention something as audacious as being pregnant when you showed up for work.

"Yep," she answered, clearly proud of herself. "I was seven months pregnant when I started."

"And the firm was fine with that?" I asked, still reeling.

"Absolutely fine. It was never an issue."

I called Paul the minute I got back from lunch. "I can have a baby and work here," I exclaimed. "I can have a baby my first year." So it was that I reported for duty more than a year later, on my first day of work, quite pregnant.

I settled into work easily. Everyone at the firm was welcoming and friendly. It was clearly going to be a nice place to work. I struck up a friendship with a colleague down the hall from me and who had just returned from maternity leave. She was happy to find a pregnant woman nearby when she came back to work. She asked me how often I was seeing the doctor. I told her how often I saw my obstetrician and my perinatologist, and she was surprised.

"Wow, that's a lot," she said. "That seems like more appointments than I had when I was seven months."

"I'm high risk," I explained. "That's why I have so many appointments."

"High risk? You?" she asked, surprised. "You don't look high risk." I love comments like that. I have been told so many times that I don't look like someone who has diabetes. Who do I look like, then?

"I have diabetes," I said

"Oh, I had diabetes when I was pregnant, too," she said. Her use of the past tense was not lost on me. She *had* diabetes. That was not a sentence I would ever be able to utter. Mine would always be the present tense. "Gestational diabetes," she clarified. Gestational diabetes is characterized by high glucose levels in a pregnant woman who does not already have diabetes. That condition, which must be monitored closely during the pregnancy, typically goes away after the baby is born.

"You did?" I asked. "Did you have to take insulin?"

"Oh no," she answered. *Nothing as drastic as that,* the tone of her voice implied. "But I did have to check my glucose level every day."

"You did?" I asked again. "How many times a day did you have to test?"

"Once a day. I had to do a glucose test every single day." Hearing this was like a kick in the stomach—unintentional—but still a kick in the stomach.

I decided to take one more shot. I needed to find a similarity between her diabetes and mine that would allow me to deduce that because her baby had been healthy, mine would be as well.

"Were your glucose levels very high?" I asked.

"Oh yes, sometimes they were," she said.

Knowing that highs are relative, I asked her, "How high was high for you?"

"Well, it was close to 130 a few times," she answered gravely. If the once-a-day glucose testing was a kick in the stomach, that response was a full body blow—unintentional once again, but a wicked blow nonetheless. Close to 130 was her high. One hundred thirty was what I hoped for as a low some days.

I needed to switch gears. The exchange had not given me the comfort I had hoped for. "How are you now?" I asked, knowing that her son was now several months old. "The diabetes, I mean. How's your diabetes now?"

"I haven't had any more issues with it. After the baby was born, I was pretty much back to normal. My doctor says I shouldn't have to worry about it, but they will check my glucose level at my annual exams from now on," she reported. Women who have had gestational diabetes are more likely than the general population to develop Type 2 diabetes later in life.

"Good for you," I said, and I meant it. I do not for an instant intend to minimize the stress and fear that a woman who has gestational diabetes must endure. For a woman who has never seen 130 on a glucose meter, the prospect of seeing that number is as disturbing to her as 330 is for me. But it is still hard to hear diabetes referred to in the past tense. It is a blessing for the person whose past it is. It is depressing for the person whose present and future it is.

18

One Saturday that fall, a bright, sunny, unseasonably warm morning, Paul shook me to wake me up. I hated being woken up that way. I needed to be eased into the day. "Amy, you're all wet. Your thighs are all wet."

"What?" I asked groggily.

"I think you're bleeding," Paul said.

I rubbed my legs together. My thighs were slick; they slipped right off each other. I reached under my nightgown and put my hand between my legs. I pulled my hand back up and looked, horrified, at my fingertips: blood. Lots of blood. "Oh, my God," I moaned. I couldn't find the breath to scream. "Where's the phone? Get me the phone." *Please, please, please* was the only thought that ran through my head. *Please, don't let this be happening. Please, please, please.*

I dialed Dr. Anderson's office without needing to look for the number. I got the answering service. It was a Saturday. The office was closed. The service told me the doctor would call me back right away. I was afraid to stand up, afraid to breathe, afraid to do anything. The doctor called me back before I even had time to work myself into a frenzy. "Go straight to the emergency room," she told me. "Don't drive. Have your husband drive you. I'll meet you there."

I was out of bed and dressed, practically before I had hung up the phone. We rushed out of the house, Paul guiding me by my elbow, as if that protective gesture could somehow help us. He heard me talking beneath my breath. "What are you saying?" he asked.

I couldn't answer him. I just kept talking, quietly, calmly, to my baby. "You're going to be okay, little baby. You're going to be fine, don't worry, little girl." I held my hard, protruding belly firmly as we drove to the hospital. It was the first day of October. I was three days shy of my 33rd birthday, sixty days shy of my due date.

If I thought years ago that being an insulin-dependent diabetic was the way to move ahead in an emergency room queue, I learned on that day one thing that trumps it: pre-term labor. Pre-term labor will get you right through any emergency-room waiting line.

Here's what had happened sometime before I awoke on that first day of October: I had gone into labor. With my baby having percolated just thirty of the forty weeks, my body was trying to force her out. Apparently I was having contractions. I couldn't even feel them. If I put my hands on my belly, I could feel the surface of my belly become unbelievably hard, as hard as a board, but I couldn't feel the contractions internally. I wasn't doubled over in pain, moaning and wailing like the many women I'd watched having babies on TV shows. I didn't even feel a cramp.

I only knew that I was having contractions because I was attached to a monitor that registered when they occurred. There were sensors on my belly, and the nurse gave me a kind of beeper, sort of like a call button. She told me that I should press the button each time I felt a contraction. They were trying to gauge how well I could feel my contractions and trying at the same time to estimate whether what I was feeling matched up with the reality of what was happening. The nurse left the room. She promised to return in fifteen to twenty minutes. I lay in my hospital bed, holding the beeper in my hands, waiting to feel a contraction. I didn't feel anything.

"You never pressed the button," the nurse said when she came back in. She was looking at a printout from the monitor I was attached to. The printout indicated when I had a contraction, and it would have also shown, had I pressed that button, when I pressed it.

"I didn't feel anything," I said

She studied the printout for a moment more, her face pointed down. She peered at me from over the rims of her glasses. "You are having a contraction every five minutes," she told me.

I was given a medication intravenously to slow and, hopefully, to stop the contractions. I stayed in the hospital bed for four days. I couldn't get out of that bed at all, for any reason. The management of my diabetes was delegated to the hospital staff. They had a schedule for when my glucose needed to be tested. It was a textbook schedule, a one-size-fits-all approach that was likely applied to all patients with diabetes: one glucose test before every meal and maybe a test before I fell asleep at night, if the night nurse had time.

That wasn't a manageable glucose-testing schedule for a pregnant woman who had Type 1 diabetes. There was no way I could manage my diabetes on three or four glucose tests a day, and there was no way I was going to take the chance of having an errant high after a meal when the staff would not be testing my glucose. I let the hospital staff test my glucose when they were instructed to—indeed, I was happy to be spared the personal expense of a few test strips a day—and then I supplemented prescribed glucose tests with my own tests, on my own meter.

The staff left it up to me to determine when I needed to take my injections of insulin and what my doses should be. A seasoned nurse had questioned me about my diabetes-treatment regimen when I was admitted to the hospital. Satisfied that I sounded like someone who was on top of the treatment, she had said to me, "Now we're going to let you tell us how much insulin you need to take and when you need to take it. You probably know that better than we do." That was a good sign. It told me that maybe some of the staff knew more about treatment of Type 1 diabetes than I had given them credit for. This woman knew that often the best person to ask how to treat a person with diabetes is the person with diabetes. I respected her for that.

Dr. Anderson came to check on me every day while I was in the hospital. Although her office was elsewhere, she had to come to that hospital most days to deliver a baby or to check on a newborn, so she would come into my room to see how I was doing. The first time she stopped by, I asked her, as I did whenever anything new or undesirable happened, "Is this because of my diabetes? Am I having early labor because of my diabetes?" Was my bad luck sign running the show again?

"It's hard to say, Amy," she answered. "It could be related. We just don't always know." Although I had only been practicing law for a few weeks at that point, I recognized her response as being as lawyerly as it was medical.

My contractions slowed to a stable rate, and I was sent home from the hospital on my birthday. I was instructed to stay in bed for four weeks. I could get up to use the bathroom, and I could take a shower every other day, but that was it. The boys were in school every day, and they needed to be dropped off, picked up, driven around to after-school activities and, of course, fed and otherwise cared for. We also had Lily, our puppy—our nearly housebroken but not-quite-out-of-the-woods puppy. That was an awful lot for one person.

Paul soldiered on admirably for a few days. Although I was in bed doing nothing, it wasn't easy for me, either. It was painful to lie in bed and listen to my household try to function without me:

"Dad, have you seen my shin guards?"

"Dad, do I have any clean khakis?"

"Dad, I'm hungry. When are we going to have dinner?"

"Has anyone seen my backpack? Oh, I just stepped in something wet. I think Lily peed."

The calls, the questions, the confusion—snippets of it all wafted up to me in our second-floor bedroom for a few hours each day, from the time when the boys got home from school until the time that they went to sleep. And there were a few that were particularly hard to overhear:

"Dad, is Amy going to be okay?"

"What'll happen if Amy has the baby now?"

"Dad, when can Amy get out of bed?"

My mother came up and helped us for a couple of weeks. I've talked about the downside of having a mother who spent most of her life working as a registered nurse in a hospital. Now let me tell you the upside: My mother can walk into any state of domestic disarray and whip it into shape in under thirty minutes.

The engine of her car had not even cooled before she had a load of laundry going, the ironing board set up, and the iron plugged in. Who knows where she found those tools in my house. Soon dinner was in the oven, and clean sheets were on my bed, which she could change without me getting out of it. The puppy had been walked and fed and was asleep, to boot, and the boys were doing their homework. On top of it all, she seemed to love every minute of it. I suppose the flip side of me having spent my whole life thinking that I needed to take care of myself was that I had a mother who wished I would sometimes need taking care of. Her wish was certainly granted.

I managed my diabetes from my bed. My bedside table held my glucose meter, logbook, insulin and syringes, and glucose pills, in case my glucose fell too low. I was still calling Dr. Landini's office every two days, as I had throughout my pregnancy. My need for insulin at that point seemed to have reached a plateau. I was still taking dramatically higher doses than I had before I was pregnant, but my need for insulin was not increasing with the regularity that it had during the several months that led up to my labor.

I had an appointment with Dr. Anderson once every week. My mother drove me to those appointments because I wasn't allowed to drive. At every one of those weekly appointments, I was attached to a fetal stress monitor that would record the baby's heartbeat. I would be left alone in the exam room with the monitor attached to my belly, and I'd listen to my baby's heartbeat bounce off the walls, the floor, the ceiling—filling up that room—for what seemed like an eternity. It always sounded to me as if her heart was beating too fast. It seemed as if she must have been in a panic. But at the end of each test, the doctor would tell me that everything sounded fine. Then I would go home and wait in my bed for another week to pass.

Finally, after I had been in bed a full month, the doctor told me I could resume my usual activities. I had reached the thirty-sixth week of my pregnancy. If the baby were to be born now, she would more than likely not face major challenges. One particular concern about a baby whose mother has Type 1 diabetes is that the baby's lungs are slow to develop. The baby's lungs at thirty weeks, when I had first gone into labor, would probably not have been sufficiently developed to let her breathe on her own. Considering that the repeated fetal stress tests I had undergone had not shown anything unusual at the thirty-six-week mark, Dr. Anderson was confident: If getting out of bed and resuming day-to-day activities caused me to go into labor, the baby should be able to handle it.

I visited the doctor for my last exam before going back to work. It was a Friday, and I was scheduled to start work again, on a reduced-hours basis, the following Monday. On my way out of the doctor's office, I stopped by the front desk to set up an appointment for the following Friday. "The doctor will be out of town next Friday," the receptionist told me. "Can we schedule you for the following Monday?"

"Sure," I said, noting the appointment on my calendar. "See you then."

19

On November 1, a Monday, one month to the day after the early labor had begun, I was sworn into the Virginia Bar. The next day I stayed at home and rested. I had returned to work on a reduced schedule and was only required to be in the office every other day. So the day after that, Wednesday, I went into the office. I didn't have any work to do at that point because I had been phased off the matters I was working on when I had been on bed rest. Until the baby came, work would be more of a social exercise than anything else. A few lawyers whose offices were near mine asked me to join them for lunch at a local chili restaurant. The restaurant was a classic dive, a Washington, D.C., institution.

"You're going to go *there*?" a secretary who worked on my hallway asked me. "You're going to go there and eat chili when you're about to have a baby?" She was honestly stunned.

"Well, sure, why not?" I asked.

"If you eat chili from that restaurant today, I'll bet you go into labor tomorrow," she said. She was smiling, but she wasn't kidding.

"I'll take my chances," I said, smiling back at her and hurrying to catch up with my colleagues.

We squeezed into a booth at the chili restaurant. Well, I suppose I was the only one who had to squeeze in. My stomach was huge, and I barely fit between the seat and table. When our chili arrived, I excused myself to go to the ladies' room. I had intentionally waited for the food to arrive, because I wanted to eyeball it before I decided how much insulin to take. The size of the serving, how much cornbread came with it, whether it had sour cream—all of that would factor into my dosage.

No one there knew I had diabetes. They assumed I was going to the bathroom to relieve my pressured bladder, not to prick my finger and then give myself a shot. I never liked to bring up the fact of my diabetes with people who didn't already know about it. For those unfamiliar with the disease, I didn't always have the energy to explain what it was all about. Many times, upon learning that I had diabetes, someone would say, "You do? But you look so healthy."

I didn't like to explain the different types of diabetes and that many people with diabetes did not have to take insulin, although I did. I didn't like explaining that I was not part of the epidemic and that I couldn't control my diabetes through diet and exercise alone. I didn't like the different way that some people treated me after they found out, always watching me to see if I might faint or require some emergency medical treatment. I didn't like always having to reassure them that I would be okay, that they weren't responsible for my well-being. And because I was pregnant, I really didn't like the way people would glimpse at my protruding belly, pretend not to have looked, and then say, "You do? Isn't that what Julia Roberts had in *Steel Magnolias?*"

With people familiar with the disease, the discussion wasn't much easier. Those familiar with Type 1 would often tell me how their uncle, their neighbor, their first-grade teacher, or someone they knew, had lost a foot to diabetes or was on dialysis or had to stop working because their eyesight had become so poor. It has always boggled my mind that people will do that. I'm sure there's some sociological theory that explains it, but I don't know what it is.

They are the same people who will look at a woman who is nine months pregnant and say, "Well, I hope your delivery is easier than mine was. I was in labor for more than twenty-four hours, and they waited too long to give me an epidural, so I couldn't take anything for the pain. After I pushed for eighteen hours, the doctor did a full episiotomy to try to get the baby out, but he was breech and just wouldn't come out, so they slapped the gas mask on me and did an emergency C-section. I didn't even see him come into this world. Sometimes I think he's not mine. I just have to take the hospital's word for it that they gave me the right baby. I don't remember a thing."

And those stories always culminate in some sort of ominous finale in which the teller's bladder control or sex life or ability to sit for long periods of time has never been the same. Great. Thanks for sharing.

And so I did not share, when I excused myself to use the ladies' room at the chili restaurant, that I was not just going there to pee. I found to my dismay that in keeping with the original charm of the restaurant, the bathroom had not been updated in many years. It was tiny. An airplane lavatory would have seemed spacious by comparison. I had to put my purse on the floor. I could no longer sit on the toilet and balance my purse and my testing supplies on my lap because I no longer had a lap.

I balanced my glucose meter on the edge of the rust-stained sink, pricked my finger, and squeezed the drop of blood onto the test strip. I waited for my glucose level to be displayed on the screen. I threw away the test strip and packed up my glucose meter. Taking a deep breath first, I bent over slowly, returned my glucose meter to my purse, and then fished around in my purse for the pouch that contained my vial of insulin and my syringes. I righted myself, and was greeted by my red-faced, puffy image in the mirror.

Look away, I told myself. I inverted the vial of insulin, filled the syringe, and then placed the glass vial carefully on the edge of the sink. Holding the syringe in my teeth, I pulled up my maternity dress, pulled down my maternity stockings, and gave myself an injection of insulin in my thigh. Then, resting the used syringe on the edge of the sink, near the vial of insulin but not close enough to upset it, I pulled my maternity stockings back up and my dress back down. I replaced the protective cover of the syringe back on the tip of the needle, careful not to re-stick myself, placed it and the vial of insulin back in their little pouch, and returned the pouch to my purse.

There's got to be a better way, I thought.

20

I would guess that the woman who predicted I would go into labor the day after eating the chili has done well in the stock market. I did go into labor the next day. That day, a Thursday, I was crampy and had a mild backache the whole day. When Paul came home from work, I told him how I felt.

"You're going to have the baby," he said. "I'll bet you have her tomorrow."

"I'm not going to have her tomorrow. She's not due for three and a half more weeks," I snapped. While it was true that the baby's actual due date was three and a half weeks away, I was scheduled to have a Caesarean section in about two weeks. My doctor preferred to deliver the baby a little early, under the controlled conditions of a planned C-section, as is often the case with babies whose mothers have diabetes.

I didn't sleep well all night. I tossed and turned. I couldn't get comfortable in any position. My stomach was hard again. I still didn't have the wailing type of pain that I like to think of as sitcom labor, but I knew from my experience the month before that I was having contractions. I tried to time them, using the very crude method of keeping my hands on my belly and watching the digital clock by our bed, marking off the minutes between when I would feel my belly harden and when it would relax. It was inexact science, to say the least, and I was also drifting in and out of sleep between contractions.

In the morning Paul took the boys to school, and I took a shower. I thought taking a shower was such a civilized and positive thing to do: taking control of the circumstances of the birth of my child, shaping our destiny. I had heard many women say that after going into labor and before going into the hospital, they had taken a shower, shaved their legs, and even painted their nails. While shaving my legs and painting my nails were activities I reserved for the postpartum phase—probably two years into the postpartum phase—I was glad to have a nice shower.

When Paul returned from dropping off the boys at school, I called my doctor's office. I needed Dr. Anderson's calm, reassuring voice. I needed to know what to do.

"The doctor is out of town until Monday," the receptionist reminded me. I had completely forgotten.

The news derailed me. What if I was in labor? Was I really going to have this baby without the doctor who had seen me through this whole pregnancy and had been my only gynecologist for my adult life—the person whose colleague had diagnosed my diabetes? My doctor was a sole practitioner. Other than Dr. Landini, who didn't deliver babies, I had not seen any other doctor over the course of my pregnancy.

"Well, what should I do?" I asked, trying to stay calm. "I think I'm in labor."

"There is another doctor covering for her at the hospital—you can call there," the receptionist told me. "Let me give you her name and beeper number." My glucose log was the only thing that I had near the telephone in my bedroom when the receptionist gave me the information, so I jotted it down in that. There, in one thick, rat-eared journal, sat page after page of the records of my glucose levels and all of the injections of insulin that I had given myself for the past thirty-some weeks. The last entry in the journal was the name and phone number of a doctor whom I'd never met but who would deliver my baby.

I was admitted immediately upon arriving at the hospital. Once again, Type 1 diabetes and pre-term labor proved to be a winning combination in the emergency-room triage line. I met the doctor who would deliver my baby as soon as I was admitted. There could not have been a better stand-in for the obstetrician whom I had known for so many years and whom I had trusted completely over the course of my high-risk pregnancy. I understood right away why Dr. Anderson would have aligned herself with this other doctor as a replacement.

To my surprise, I was already three centimeters dilated, but I still was experiencing no discernible pain. When the doctor checked me an hour later, I was five centimeters dilated. Still I had no pain. Perhaps the lack of pain was some sort of karmic retribution for my efforts over the past thirty-six weeks. *Give the poor woman a break this afternoon, she's done a good job,* the gods might have been thinking.

"Alright, we're going to get you ready," the doctor said. "You're going to have a baby in the next couple of hours."

We agreed that I should have a Caesarean section. The doctor gave me the option of laboring and trying for a vaginal delivery, but there was always the wild card of what my glucose level would do during labor and delivery. Not knowing that I would be having a baby that day, I had taken my normal dose of long-acting insulin when I woke up in the morning, and that insulin would be working in my system for many hours.

The energy required to labor and deliver a baby obviate the need for insulin. A woman burns enough glucose in this exercise to compensate for any need for insulin. I had been told but could not really let myself believe that a woman with Type 1 diabetes may not need any insulin at all for several days following delivery, because her body continues to burn glucose to make up for the energy expended during labor and delivery. The fact that I had already taken insulin that day, coupled with the strain that I would undergo during labor and delivery, argued in favor of a C-section.

I had not taken a childbirth class. I had not read about the eighth month and beyond in any of my "what to expect" guides to pregnancy. Things seemed to get a little scary after the eighth month, and I wasn't sure how the additional knowledge would do anything other than give me something new to worry about. The one time that I had mustered the courage to read about a vaginal delivery, the tale ended with a doctor leaving a surgical sponge inside a woman's uterus. When he realized his error, he reached back in up to his elbow, as if he were fishing around in a shopping bag, to retrieve it. *That*, I thought, *is not something I need to know about.* I reasoned that, God willing, my baby was going to be born, whether or not I knew all of the possibilities of what could go wrong, so I would rather go into it blindly.

The doctor was delighted, if not more than a little surprised, when I confessed to having no real idea what was about to happen. "You haven't taken a childbirth class? You don't have a birthing plan?" She threw back her head and laughed. "Oh, thank goodness. You're not going to be telling me what to do. And you're a lawyer, too." I gathered from her comment that lawyers don't always make the best patients. Lawyers probably read everything there is to read and then take any opportunity to proffer their opinions about what the doctor should do in an area wholly outside of the lawyer's area of expertise. She placed her hand affectionately on my leg. "Oh, I like you. I really like you," she said, still laughing.

The first step in the C-section process, I learned in real time, is for the anesthesiologist to calibrate the dosage for the epidural. I would be fully awake and cognizant while the baby was surgically removed from my uterus, but by virtue of an epidural anesthesia block, I would be numb from the chest down. Before the actual surgical procedure was performed, the anesthesiologist would give me a "practice" dose to see if the numbing effect was sufficient. The anesthesia was injected, and I lay in my hospital bed waiting for it to take effect. Before long, my legs began to feel tingly. Then they were numb. Soon I couldn't feel them at all, nor could I move them.

While I waited for the anesthesiologist to return, I decided I should do a glucose test. We were getting down to the wire, and I hadn't checked my glucose level in a while. The insulin I had taken that morning would still be acting, and I hadn't been allowed to eat anything during the past few hours while I was being prepped for surgery. I pricked my finger and waited for the beep: 79. Heavy sigh. Seventy nine was not going to get me through the next half hour, much less a C-section. I rang the call button, and a nurse appeared in my room moments later.

"I have a low glucose level," I explained to her. "I'm not sure what to do. I'm not supposed to eat anything, so I don't think I can have any glucose pills. But I need something."

"What is your glucose level?" she asked.

I reported the 79 to her.

She referred to a chart in her file and then said, "You're fine. As long as your glucose level is above 70, you're fine." She turned and started to leave the room.

"Wait," I said, and she stopped at the door. "I'm not fine. My glucose level will be below 70 in about ten minutes if I don't do something about it now. And it will be below 60 ten minutes after that. I'm crashing. I'm about to have a C-section, and I'm crashing." I was frightened. A cookie-cutter reading of my glucose level by someone clearly unfamiliar with Type 1 diabetes was not going to help me now. I knew what I needed. I needed glucose. I just didn't know how to get it.

Before the nurse had a chance to respond to me, a commanding voice behind her said, "Listen to her." Though I couldn't see her, I knew it was the doctor. "Listen to this patient. She's an insulin-dependent diabetic. She took insulin this morning, and she's about to go into surgery. If she is telling you her glucose level is crashing, get her some glucose. Now. The last thing we need is for her to lose consciousness."

The nurse scurried away, and moments later a bag of glucose and an intravenous line were wheeled into my room. I was then connected intravenously to the glucose. My glucose level was not going fall too low during the C-section. The doctor winked at me and smiled.

I was wheeled into the operating room, Paul at my side. What happened next seems in my recollection to have been so quick and easy that only the result deserves retelling. After what seemed like only five minutes on the operating room table, I met my daughter, Emily. She was there, with me, and she could breathe. The size of her head was normal. The length of her arms and legs was normal. Her spine was normal. She was six pounds, ten ounces of pure, baby-girl perfection. I thought I would never see that day.

The doctor closed my incision, a nurse cleaned up my daughter, and they wheeled both of us back to my hospital room. I couldn't believe I was holding her in my arms, and she was no longer inside of me. I couldn't believe she was really healthy.

We were just getting situated back in our room when a team of medical professionals arrived, consulting a file. "Your baby is fine, but her glucose level is low," one of them told me.

"What?" I asked "How low? How do you know her glucose level?"

"We tested it after she was born. Her glucose level was 57," the same person told me without any real sense of urgency.

I had been told to expect this. Often the baby of a mother who has Type 1 diabetes has a low glucose level when she is born. That's because her little pancreas has been pumping out extra insulin to compensate for any high glucose levels she was receiving from her mother. So I shouldn't have been surprised, but just hearing a glucose level of 57 scared the wits out of me. I was also confused about when she had been tested. How had they pricked her tiny little finger?

"We didn't prick her finger. We pricked her heel. Here, look," the person said, reaching to the baby who was in my arms, unwrapping the swaddling blanket and showing me her foot, which was wrapped in gauze. Poor little thing, I thought, only a few minutes in this world and already she had felt pain.

"Well, 57," I said, snapping out of it. "What do you do about that? Do you give her glucose?" I was looking down at her sweet little face, not at the doctor, during this whole conversation. Nothing could be wrong with her. It just couldn't be.

"We'll bring you some formula to give her," he told me. "And then we'll check her again in a few hours."

A bottle of formula arrived straightaway. I lifted my baby a little bit in my arms, angling her head higher. I tilted the bottle of formula and eased the nipple against her little pursed mouth. Her eyes were closed. They didn't open in response to the bottle, but her mouth did. Her little mouth opened slightly, and she made the smallest, nearly imperceptible, sucking movement. I slid the tip into her mouth, and she drank some of the formula. *Drink, baby, drink,* I beseeched her silently. *We need to get your glucose level up, and then you are going to be just fine.*

We continued that way for a few days. I would give Emily an ounce or so of formula every few hours, and the hospital staff would come by to prick her heel and get her glucose level. The procedure always culminated with a big, gauzy bow being tied around her foot. On the fourth day, after she'd had several glucose test results in a normal and stable range, the doctor told me that they wouldn't need to check her glucose level any more. She was fine. She was out of the woods. Her pancreas had regulated her insulin secretion to match the glucose level in her body, not the glucose level in her diabetic mother's body.

"When should I have her checked again?" I asked, not understanding that it was really over.

"When she's 55," the doctor said.

I looked him in the eye, afraid to believe what he had said. "Really?" I asked.

"Really," he said, smiling.

PART III

21

Burnout. It happens to us all. Kids burn out on school. Adults burn out on work. Parents burn out on parenting. And people who have diabetes, all types of diabetes, burn out on managing it.

Diabetes burnout is a well-documented phenomenon. Books have been written on the subject. Anyone who lives with this disease in any of its forms knows that it's easier many days to let things slide than to manage it closely. Particularly for people who take insulin and whose diabetes therefore requires a nearly constant level of awareness, the urge to loosen up on it all can be hard to resist. It's easy to skip a few finger pricks; easy to scarf down a snack without injecting any insulin; easy to let your glucose run high so you don't have to worry about it for a few hours, or better yet, a few days.

My diabetes burnout didn't happen overnight. It didn't happen right after I had the baby, but gradually, over time, it accumulated. It festered insidiously.

When I had been pregnant, I had a very specific, tremendously important motivation for controlling my diabetes on a daily, even on an hourly basis. The time period for the tight control was finite. After those forty weeks—or thirty-six, as it turned out—I could loosen up a little. At that point, I had lived with diabetes for only about three and a half years. It was a little early for me to burn out. Three and a half years is nothing in the lifetime of a person with diabetes. Try ten years. Try fifteen. Now we're getting into the burnout years.

After Emily was born and she was enrolled in day care and I was back at work, after life picked up its typically frenzied pace, it was very easy to start to let my diabetes management slide. After there was no life other than mine at stake—and no one else would suffer the effects of poor control, and even those would likely be many years in the future—it was all the easier.

I grew weary of so many aspects of keeping up with this disease: weary of having enough glucose test strips on hand for ten to twelve glucose tests per day, weary of keeping up with my never-ending need for syringes. After Emily was born, I wasn't able to go back to my pre-pregnancy regimen of three shots per day.

I had started to see a new endocrinologist. Dr. Landini had been my diabetes specialist only during my pregnancy, and the new doctor had me stay on the four-shots-a-day protocol that Dr. Landini had started, though at much lower doses than when I was pregnant. On bad days I might need to have a couple of extra injections if I had any unusual highs throughout the day or at bedtime, bringing the total to five or six shots per day.

The logistics of using five or six new syringes each day were daunting, to say the least. Doing the math and running conservative averages, this comes out to about thirty-five syringes per week, around 150 per month. I ordered my syringes in boxes of hundreds, yet still I never seemed to have enough. I had syringes in my bathroom, in my kitchen, in my purse, in Emily's diaper bag, in my brief case, in my desk drawers, in the glove box of the car.

It was hard to tell which syringes were used, and which were new. You can't just throw a syringe into the trash can after using it. There are disposal requirements, and so I would end up with huge stock-piles of syringes that I had used when there was no place to dispose of them. In my office, for example, I had an entire desk drawer full of used syringes. When I was pregnant and out of the office on bed rest, and then later out on maternity leave, a temporary attorney was assigned to use my office. When I heard that someone would be in my office, sitting at my desk, I called one of my friends at work and asked, "Can you do me a favor? Can you stop by and see who's using my office? And can you please tell that person that I'm not a drug addict but that I have diabetes? Tell them that's why I have a drawer full of syringes."

Every few months I emptied my desk drawer into a Macy's shopping bag and brought the used syringes home to dispose of them properly. On those days I'd be nervous that someone in the elevator might be curious about what had been on sale at Macy's that day, what was in the bag. I guarded the bag closely. The times that I came home with my big bag of used-up syringes, I usually had a pretty good shot at getting some sympathy from Paul.

The drama that had surrounded my first shot so many years ago had long since disappeared. The sadness about my condition had dried up as well. No one, not the person with diabetes and not the family members who love the person with diabetes, can suffer over every single shot. The shots become so routine that neither the person with diabetes nor the family members pause when they occur. I could be cooking dinner, helping the boys with their homework, and giving Emily a bottle, and in between the stove, the fridge, and the homework table I would swing by the kitchen counter, prick my finger, pull out a syringe, sink it into a vial of insulin, withdraw my dose, and inject myself before anyone even had time to notice what I was doing.

So the routine of so many insulin injections becomes, well, routine. Nobody notices a thing. Each individual injection is a one-time, forgettable event. You see it for a few seconds, then it's over and done with, and everyone moves on until the next one a few hours later.

It's quite a different experience, however, to see the accumulated pile of weeks' and months' worth of multiple daily injections. A shopping bag full of syringes is quite a powerful statement. It says, *Okay, maybe the injections are only given one at a time, but just look how they pile up. Just look at how many shots this person has given herself. And those were only the shots at work. Those weren't the shots at home; they weren't the shots before bedtime; they weren't the shots on the weekend.* A shopping bag of used syringes packs quite a wallop.

The first time Paul saw the contents of my big brown Macy's bag, he came as close as he ever has to shedding a few tears in sympathy. But better than crying, he cooked dinner that night. After that, a shopping bag full of syringes was usually good for a dinner or maybe even a load of laundry.

Another logistical issue, another factor contributing to my building sense of burnout, was that having to do so many injections in a day made it hard sometimes to keep track of whether or not I had given myself one. I was usually pretty good about knowing whether I'd done each pre-meal shot of short-acting insulin. It was always the last thing I did right before I sat down to eat. After I had everyone's food on the table, I would slip back into the kitchen to give myself a shot to cover the meal. I preferred to wait until right before the meal for a couple of reasons. I could never be sure until I was actually sitting down and eating whether I would be eating any meal on schedule. There was always the chance that at the last minute I would get a call from work that I had to take or one of the kids would remember that he needed to be driven somewhere, and before I knew it my meal would be postponed for another hour or so.

It also was easier to estimate how many grams of carbohydrates I was eating if I waited until my meal was ready and on my plate. The dosage of short-acting insulin that I injected before each meal varied, depending on how many carbohydrates I would consume. It was often not until I had actually served myself and had seen what was on my plate that I knew roughly how much insulin to take. So my pre-meal shots were pretty easy to keep up with.

The shot of long-acting insulin was a bit harder to track. Rather than doing a long-acting shot first thing in the morning, as I had for the first few years after my diagnosis, I'd switched after my pregnancy to a new long-acting form of insulin that I injected before bed each night. Talk about a leap of faith. Telling a person with diabetes to inject a syringe-full of insulin and then go to bed and fall asleep requires a huge leap of faith. Lows during sleep are what we fear most.

But I did it. As with so many other things during the course of this disease, I followed the instructions of my physicians, shut my eyes, jumped in, and hoped for the best.

But it was hard to remember, many nights, whether I'd given myself the bedtime shot. I would put on my pajamas, wash my face, brush my hair, floss and brush my teeth, crawl into bed, and then not be able to remember whether I had done the shot that I needed to get me through the next twenty-four hours. It's like when you get in bed and then lie awake wondering if you had turned off the iron or the oven. It's easy to get up and check the iron or the oven. It's not so easy to confirm whether you gave yourself a shot. Usually I would start by nudging Paul and asking him, "Did I do a shot before I came to bed?"

"Yes," he'd answer. He always answered yes. Just as he always answers yes when I ask him if the doors are locked. He just wants to go to sleep. He always thinks everything is fine.

"How do you know?" I would press, knowing that he hadn't given it any real thought.

If he said, "I saw you do it," and then was able to give some identifying particulars, such as where I was when I did the shot, whether or not I said "Ouch," and so forth, I'd be satisfied.

If he clearly was fudging and actually had no idea whether I'd done my shot, he'd say something like, "Well, I didn't see you do it, if that's what you want to know. But come on, it's you. You always do your shot. You'd never forget." With that, he would roll over and go to sleep. I would be left staring at the ceiling, trying to reconstruct in minute detail the events of the half hour or so before I had gone to bed. Based on that reconstruction, I would make an educated guess about whether I had done my shot, and then I would weigh the risk of missing a shot versus possibly giving myself two injections of my bedtime insulin. Two injections of my bedtime insulin could be lethal. Somehow, in so many years of bedtime injections, I had never made that mistake.

So a big part of what contributed to my lax approach to managing my diabetes, and a lot of what was leading to the burnout, were the logistical challenges of keeping up with it all. Keeping up with the test strips. Keeping up with the syringes. Keeping up with how many shots I had done. Keeping up with all of that, on top of everything else I had to keep up with in my life. Who wouldn't want a break from all that?

Apart from the logistics of keeping up with the supplies, I was tired of worrying about lows. I found myself letting my glucose level run too high too often so that I wouldn't have to worry about the possibility of going too low. I couldn't manage my busy life and keep my diabetes tightly controlled. In the mornings I let my glucose level run too high because I didn't want to be low when I was taking the kids to school or when I was driving myself to work. During the days, I let it run too high if I had a meeting or a long conference call, or on the chance I would be called unexpectedly into another attorney's office. In the late afternoon and evenings, I let it run too high so that I didn't have to worry about a low when I was driving home or racing to pick up a kid from practice or to watch a Little League game. On the weekends, I let it run too high so that I could run around to the dry cleaner, the grocery store, the soccer field, the post office, without having to prick my finger between each stop.

I was years into my disease, and the burnout was getting the upper hand. It was making my days a little easier but my long-term prospects a little bleaker.

22

I got an e-mail today that broke my heart. It aches deeply, in several different places, for a fourteen-year-old girl whom I never knew. My heart aches in the place where I am a mother, in the place where I was once a teenage girl, and finally, in the place where I'm still a person with diabetes, afraid to fall asleep many nights. My heart aches so much that I think I will never quite forget this. I hope I don't. No one should ever forget what I am about to tell you.

The e-mail was from my friend Delia, the outreach coordinator for the Washington, D.C., chapter of the Juvenile Diabetes Research Foundation (JDRF). Just about the best thing that has come from me having diabetes is that I have gotten to know her. She's a breath of fresh air in a fairly sad community. She herself is a member of that community, another adult diagnosed with Type 1 diabetes when she was in her twenties.

After any interaction with Delia, you emerge a better person. I leave every encounter with her feeling ten years younger, ten pounds lighter, and a whole lot happier. Perhaps that's why the Capitol Chapter of the JDRF tapped her to be the person who welcomes newly diagnosed children and their families into the fold. She sends them a care package. She talks to the kids. She calms the parents.

Delia lives and breathes diabetes. It is her day job and her night life, her toil and her recreation. It isn't easy to do what she does. The burnout rate is high. But Delia doesn't burn out. She soldiers on. She does it because she loves the children. She loves them with all her heart.

Last summer Delia participated in a 100-mile bike ride to raise money for research into the causes and treatment of Type 1 diabetes.

It was no small feat to train for the event when she routinely works sixty-hour weeks and when she struggles with the challenges that all people with Type 1 diabetes have in regulating their glucose levels in a strenuous exercise program. But Delia did it. She did it because she wanted to have a goal, she wanted to reach that goal, and she wanted to raise money for diabetes research.

Delia sent me, and all of the people who donated funds for her ride, a photograph taken at the finish line of her and Jonah, a little boy who was diagnosed with Type 1 diabetes when he was two years old. Jonah was grinning from ear-to-ear. "From me and my friend Jonah!" the card read.

Delia wasn't going to do the ride again. She felt a little guilty, as anyone with her sense of commitment would, but it all had been too much: too much time, too much to try to squeeze in on top of her full-time job, and too much work to raise the $3,000 that was required to fund the ride. We had lunch in January, and she told me that. Delia and I had talked about "dead-in-bed" syndrome at that lunch, too. The name is almost too much to bear. Dead in bed. Taken, in your most vulnerable state. Taken, when you cannot fight back.

Dead-in-bed syndrome is a phenomenon in which an otherwise healthy person with diabetes, most often a teenager, is found dead in the morning after an apparently undisturbed sleep. The cause is unknown. It may be hypoglycemia. It may be cardiac arrhythmia. There's no sign of a struggle. There's no evidence of an attempt to reach out to the bedside table for a bottle of glucose pills. There are no twisted bed sheets that might indicate a seizure. The bed sheets aren't damp. There is nothing but calm. Dead calm.

Delia had been reading about dead-in-bed syndrome because it was relevant to her job. We talked about how unbelievably depressing it was to contemplate this possibility. We talked about how terrifying it was, particularly for her, a young woman living alone. But we also laughed our heads off, because she told me she had recently gotten an e-mail from someone who had said,

"Delia—Here is a really good article about dead-in-bed that I thought you might enjoy."

"What? A good article about dead-in-bed? To enjoy?" We howled. We didn't laugh because it was funny. Dear God, it certainly wasn't funny. We laughed because it was gallows humor. In truth, it was the only outlet for our terror—the sheer terror, the jolt down the spine at knowing that this syndrome is out there, and that we are in the class of people that it strikes.

That was the last I had heard from Delia until I got the e-mail from her today, saying that she was doing the ride again. And here is why, in her own words:

> I was not sure I was going to be able to participate in the JDRF Ride again this year. "Life" was in the way, and I had a busy schedule planned for the summer. A few months ago, on a cold February day, this decision changed in the blink of an eye. I was sitting in the pew of a chapel, celebrating the life of a beautiful, amazing, full of life, 14-year-old girl who died from complications of Type 1. Her blood sugar dropped too low in her sleep, and she never woke up.

I thought of the girl's parents. They must have been so tired. They'd probably set their alarm every night and woken up at 3 a.m. for the past twelve years. Each night, just hours after the parents had fallen asleep, they would've dragged themselves out of bed, gotten out the glucose meter, inserted the test strip, and fished around under the covers to find their sweet baby's fingers. Her fingers would've been chubby when she was little. There would've been dirt under the nails. But her fingers were probably long and thin now, maybe with polish on the nails. Maybe it was silly polish, teenage-girl polish— bright blue with while polka dots. But her parents could just about see, in her fingers, the young woman she would become. She was going to be an extraordinary young woman. They could see in those calloused fingertips, on the flip side of those hopelessly optimistic nails, that her lifetime of vigilance in the care of her diabetes would not be for nothing.

Their girl would've been so used to being poked and prodded that she wouldn't even wake up when they pierced the skin of her fingertip and the blood bubbled out. They'd pray for a number above 100. They might hope for one even higher, damn the long-term consequences, if they could just have a number that would give them enough peace to sleep for the next few hours. Just to see her at breakfast in the morning. Cranky or not. Homework done or not. Just as long as she would wake up.

And then one day she does not wake up. One morning, after a night like any other, she is gone. It's all over. The diabetes is over. Their daughter's life is over. Their life is over, but somehow they must live and breathe without her. She's simply gone.

I can barely type the words, because who can imagine it? Who can bear it? Waking up, pouring your coffee, taking your shower, and then going to roust your beautiful eighth-grade girl: your girl who has been so brave; your girl whose finger has been stabbed ten times a day since she was in training pants; your girl who now hides her insulin pump under her clothes so she won't look different to the other kids at middle school. Your girl who never complained about anything, who loved her life, who had everything to look forward to—and who didn't deserve to die.

23

"Hi, Ms. Ryan. This is Dr. Starr. I have your test results back. Your A1C is up a little more again. You really should think about the pump, like I mentioned in the office. Call me if you want to talk about it."

I was at my desk in my office when I saw Dr. Starr's call come in on my caller ID. I intentionally didn't answer the call. I didn't want to hear what I knew he had to say. I knew my A1C would be up. I knew he wanted me to start on an insulin pump. I decided to let his call ring through to voicemail. I'd play back the message later.

My A1Cs had stayed in a good range for several years after Emily was born. Then gradually they began to creep up. It's easy to ignore a few tenths of a percentage point increase in an A1C. I have the test done every twelve weeks, so a minor increase after such a short interval can sometimes be ignored. What's harder to ignore is the cumulative effect of all those little increases. A two-tenths of a point increase over a twelve-week period is not necessarily cause for alarm. Another three-tenths of a point increase over the next twelve weeks, in itself, may not be cause for alarm, either. If you look back just twelve weeks to your last A1C, it doesn't look like much of a jump. But if you look back further, to your A1C six months ago, one year ago, eighteen months ago, the increase is bigger. It's much easier to see and much harder to ignore.

"Why don't you think about the pump?" Dr. Starr, my new endocrinologist, had asked me at my last appointment. He was the latest in a string of about five endocrinologists whom I had seen since Dr. Landini. All the others had come up short. They didn't ask me the right questions. I was an informed patient by that point, and I knew what they should ask. If they didn't cover the right issues, I never went back. Dr. Starr turned out to be the one I would stick with. He was the one whose front office never changed, whose nurse never changed, who could always fit me in, who called personally with lab results, who always took as much time at our appointments as I needed. He remembered who my kids were, what my job was. His profession was his calling.

This wasn't the first time Dr. Starr had asked me to consider an insulin pump. He had mentioned it to me at each of my appointments for the past year or so. Though I knew a little about the pump, he explained it to me more fully.

Insulin pumps at that time had three principal features, all of which were attached to the body: an infusion set, a flexible tube (also called a "cannula"), and the pump itself. The infusion set consisted of a needle that injects a tiny plastic tube beneath the skin. The needle retracts, it doesn't remain under the skin. Only the plastic tube remains under the skin. The tube is secured in place, typically on the abdomen, by an adhesive patch. The tube, which can be several inches long, connects to a device about the size of a cell phone that contains insulin. This device is what is known as the "pump." Because traditional pumps have to remain attached to the tube that's inserted under the user's skin, the pump must remain tethered to the user. Most "pumpers," as they call themselves, attach their pumps beeper-style to their waistband or to a belt.

The pump is designed to mimic the function of a normal pancreas. Like a functional pancreas, the pump secretes a constant low dose of insulin throughout the day and night. The insulin flows at a continuous rate from the pump, through the tube, and is released under the skin of the user. This is known as the "basal" rate. The basal rate gives the user a baseline level of insulin to keep her glucose level stable round the clock but does not cover any food that the user might consume. It's the rough equivalent of the long-acting dose of insulin I took before bed each night.

When a pumper eats, she programs the pump to give her what is known as a "bolus" of insulin. The bolus dose is calculated based on the grams of carbohydrates that the user will consume and is designed to deliver an amount of insulin appropriate to cover that amount of carbohydrates. The bolus is the equivalent of the short-acting shot that I did before meals and at other times when my glucose level was too high.

People who have diabetes and use insulin pumps no longer have to give themselves shots of insulin. The pump is the sole source of insulin. When you do a bolus, the tube from the pump that's under your skin simply releases the extra insulin. You don't need to do a new shot to get the insulin; it comes through the tube that is fused to your body. You still have to test your glucose levels, but the need for a seemingly endless supply of syringes can become a thing of the past. Trying to find an injection site on your body that's not bruised and sore can become a thing of the past. Remembering whether or not you've given yourself a shot can become a thing of the past. Giving yourself an injection in a dirty, cramped stall of a public restroom can become a thing of the past.

Yet despite all the advantages of pump therapy that Dr. Starr explained to me, I couldn't be sold on the idea of the pump. I was an old dog in the diabetes world, and this was a new trick. At that time my routine of treating my diabetes with multiple daily injections was still working relatively well. My A1Cs were creeping up, but they were still in a relatively safe range. I told myself I could keep living with the inconvenience of the syringes so long as my A1Cs stayed in that range.

24

During the summer when she was thirty-nine years old and her daughters were six and four years old, my sister Betsy found two lumps in her left breast. A friend of hers at work had been diagnosed with early-stage breast cancer, and the friend had waged a campaign in the workplace to urge women to perform breast self-exams. My sister had examined herself that evening, the very day she got the message. The hard, pea-sized lumps that she felt were unmistakable.

After several excruciating days, she learned that the lumps were malignant. Several days and several procedures later, it was determined that the cancer that had been found in her breast had spread to her lymph nodes.

She and I sat in her living room, looking at the web on our laptops, paging through book after book, trying to find a life-expectancy statistic that would work for her. We found fairly good statistics for three years.

"No, three years is not long enough. Jessie will only be nine, and Lauren will only be seven," Betsy said, referring to her daughters. "That's not going to work."

"You're right, let's find another one," I agreed.

There was a somewhat encouraging statistic for five years. "Five years," she said, calculating in her head how old her daughters would be in five years. "Jessie will be eleven, and Lauren will be nine." She considered this for a moment. "No, that's not going to work, either. Just think how busy they'll be then. I can't leave David with all that." So she rejected five years as her prognosis as well.

"Should we look at ten years?" I asked hesitantly. The statistics for ten years weren't quite as encouraging.

"Ten years... let's see, Jessie will be sixteen, and Lauren will be fourteen." She barely even paused to consider this option. "Nope. That's definitely not going to work. I have to be around when they're teenagers. Do you remember how I was as a teenager? David can't cope with that alone. Can you imagine?"

During the course of our conversation, as we paged through statistic after statistic, Betsy began to formulate her strategy for dealing with her disease. Her strategy would be to live her life. No actuarial chart was going to tell her that she wouldn't be around to see her girls through their teenage years and beyond. No amount of time would ever be enough.

She wondered whether she should tell her daughters that she could die from her cancer. She asked one of her oncologists for an opinion on this. The oncologist said, "Yes, you need to prepare your daughters for that possibility."

"Don't you think that's crazy?" she asked me. "Why would I tell them that? Why would I tell them that I might die?"

I listened, not sure what to say, not sure where she was going with this.

"I could die tomorrow," she went on. "You could die tomorrow." Not exactly what I wanted to hear, but of course she was right. "Anyone could die tomorrow. So if I didn't have cancer, should I tell them when they get on the bus in the morning: 'Remember, I might get in a car accident and die today. But have a good day.'"

I had to laugh at the morbidity of it.

"'Daddy could die, too,'" she went on. "'If we're still alive, we'll see you after school. But don't worry—have a great day.'"

We were both laughing by then. Or maybe we were both crying. It was hard to tell the difference. We were both feeling the anguish of knowing that it could all be yanked out from under us at any moment. Cancer or not. Diabetes or not. Was that funny or was it sad? It was a little of the former and a lot of the latter. It was also too much to think about for long.

When I was diagnosed with diabetes, I thought I knew what was going to kill me. Diabetes was going to kill me. I was young then. I'm not young now. I'm old enough to know, as Betsy and I had laughed and cried about, that I don't know what will ultimately be my demise. I don't know what's going to kill me. Some days I think I'll be lucky if it is the diabetes that gets me. That will probably mean that I've lived a very long life.

Paul had pointed out to me, as I lay soaking in the bathtub one night before getting on a flight to the West Coast, that I'm more likely to die from slipping in the bathtub than from a plane crash—which is one of my big, irrational fears. He has also been known to remind me when I leave for work, in my car, that I'm more likely to die in a car accident on the beltway than by a terrorist strike in Washington, D.C.—which was another of my big, irrational fears in the wake of the 2001 terrorist attacks. I've mentioned to Paul that if he wants these messages to have their desired reassuring effect, he needs to work on the timing and context of when he delivers them—not in the bathtub and not when I'm getting into my car.

So, like everyone else, I don't know what's going to get me. But I do know one thing that's trying. I do know for certain one thing I'm up against. There's a lot I can't protect against—indeed most things I can't protect against—but there's one thing that I can. Maybe knowing that can help me fight the burnout. Maybe seeing my sister fight her battle would help me find a new way to fight mine.

Betsy and her family visited us the Thanksgiving after she found out she had cancer. She had no hair. She had no breasts. Yet her spirit was intact. Despite it all, she found so much to be thankful for on that holiday.

"But how are *you* doing?" she asked me. "How's the diabetes?"

"Well, not so great, sis," I began. I filled her in on the creeping A1Cs. I told her I was up to five or six shots of insulin per day. I told her I was so tired of it all. I told her about the pump—and why I was reluctant to try it.

"The pump sounds cool," she said. "Why don't you try it? You should try it."

My reasons for not wanting to try the pump were mostly superficial. I didn't want to be tethered to the beeper-like device. The reality of having a tube coming out of my body and attaching to a piece of hardware did not appeal to me at all. I didn't want to have the device affixed to my waistband for the whole world to see. If I didn't have a waistband—say if I were wearing a one-piece dress—I didn't want to worry about where I would stash the pump.

And what would I do with the pump when I needed to use the bathroom? Or when I was at the beach? Or when I took a shower? How could I roll over in bed—where I was often flanked by Paul on one side and, by daybreak, Emily on the other, with the dog usually piling in too, at some point—if I had a tube and a beeper attached to me?

The next time I saw Dr. Starr, I asked him these questions. He explained that for some of these situations, the tube could be disconnected from the infusion set and taken off with the pump for short periods of time. This would take care of showering, swimming, and maybe a few other activities. He also explained that there were lots of ways to wear the pump other than affixing it to your waistband. There was a whole line of pump fashion accessories: slips with a special hidden pocket for the pump, bras with a pocket for the pump in between the cups, pajamas with a special pump compartment, garter grips to hold the pump on the calf or thigh.

Still, one big question lurked in my mind. How were Paul and I supposed to have any kind of a sex life if I had a tube coming out of my body and a pump device attached to that?

I could talk to Dr. Starr about my kidneys. I could talk to him about my heart, my eyes, my feet. I could collect twenty-four hours' worth of urine in a jug and look him in the eyes as I handed it over to him. I could talk to him about my anxiety over lows. But to talk to him about sex was another thing altogether. Sex was not a subject that my diabetes had ever given us reason to broach. Sex was one area of my life, perhaps the only one, that diabetes hadn't changed forever. I wasn't willing to hand that one off to my disease.

"Well, there's something I've wondered about... about the pump, I mean," I stammered. I'd decided to barrel ahead, to ask Dr. Starr my question, to put it on the table.

The doctor looked at me attentively, eyebrows raised, waiting for my question. Dr. Starr has a very earnest face. In his face, you can tell exactly what he looked like when he was four years old. You can tell that he had been a cute little boy.

"What would I do with the pump when I'm... um... intimate?" I asked, using a euphemism I don't think I'd ever used before.

His eyes squinted slightly and his brow furrowed. "Do you mean—" Then his voice trailed off. He wasn't going to be the first one to say it.

"I mean when I have sex," I blurted out. There, I'd said it. What a relief. "What would I do with the pump when my husband and I have sex?"

He seemed a bit surprised. It didn't appear that he had ever been asked this question. He thought for a moment and then said, "Well, I guess you could just clip it to the bed sheet."

I had my answer. It was an answer that made me certain that the pump wouldn't work for me. I wasn't going to be condemned to a sex life that required a bed sheet to be nearby. This wouldn't work. Paul and I often sacrificed location for timing, comfort for opportunity. Our sex didn't always happen in a bed or anywhere else that would be handy to clip an insulin pump. The doctor's response also meant that I'd still have the tube coming out of my body and connecting to the pump during the act. I couldn't imagine that any tube attached to my abdomen while we were in *flagrante delicto* would remain intact. At best, it would become as twisted as a pretzel. At worst, it could dislodge and come unplugged from the pump, cutting off my insulin supply.

"But couldn't it come undone or unplugged or whatever?" I asked the doctor, referring to the tube.

He thought for a moment more. "You could always disconnect it first, and then re-connect afterwards," he suggested. He meant that I could disconnect the tube from the infusion set—the adhesive patch that remains on the body and holds in place the tube that stays under the skin—enjoy my time with my husband and then get up afterward and re-connect the tube and the pump. I would have to put on pajamas at that point, too, so I would have something to clip the pump to once I was reconnected. So much for spontaneity. So much for drifting off to a peaceful, naked sleep afterwards.

I'd just about convinced myself that high A1C or not, I wasn't going to give up this last untouched area of my life, when Dr. Starr said something that I wasn't prepared to hear. "There's a new pump you might want to think about. It doesn't have a tube outside your body. It's essentially wireless. It's just a pod that adheres to your body."

And there went my last excuse.

25

It's hard not knowing many people who have Type 1 diabetes. I know some now. I didn't know any then. The first person whom I heard about was someone I didn't know at all but who I felt was a longtime friend: Mary Tyler Moore. As a girl growing up in the 1970s, I had no greater aspiration than to be like Mary Tyler Moore. Or, more accurately, I wanted to be like Mary Richards, whom I knew far more about than I did about the actress who played her. Whichever Mary she was, I now had something in common with her.

Why did it make me feel better to learn that Mary Tyler Moore had diabetes? I think it was because I'd never known that she had it. I had watched her for hours and hours on television, and she didn't seem like someone who had a disease. She didn't seem like someone who was going to die. Or someone who was tragic. She seemed so normal. Fabulous beyond compare, but still normal.

After I was diagnosed, I used to think that there was always going to be something just a little sad about me—like an aura. I thought that people would think, maybe even murmur among themselves when I was on the other side of the room, "Oh, there's Amy, she had so much going for her. It's really a shame about the diabetes," with the implicit suggestion that it was all over for me. I thought I could never again be 100 percent happy. I was probably still going to be really, really happy sometimes, like I used to be, maybe somewhere in the high 90s percentage-wise, but there was always going to be this cloud of my lifelong disease to add an air of sadness to who I am and to what others thought of me.

But there was nothing sad about Mary Tyler Moore. She was doing the same thing I was doing every day of her life—checking her glucose levels frequently, hanging on from injection to injection—and I had never known it. There was not even a hint of sadness about Mary Tyler Moore. If Mary could do it, perhaps I could do it, too.

A few years later, when I was farther into my life with this disease, and it was still rare to run across someone who shared it, Paul and the boys called me excitedly into the family room one evening. They were watching television, flipping channels, and they had stumbled upon the Miss America pageant. I rounded the corner into the family room and was met with the glowing smile of a beautiful, poised brunette on the screen.

"Wow, she's pretty," I said.

"But guess what? She has diabetes—and it's your kind." The boys were so excited. They were so happy to tell me this news. There's not often much good breaking news to tell a person who has diabetes. You'd like to be the person who tells your wife or tells your stepmother, "Hey, I've got some great news about diabetes." That opportunity doesn't present itself often, but this was pretty darn close. This was fantastic news. Nicole Johnson, a young woman with Type 1 diabetes, was about to be crowned Miss America. I had chills. *How can she be on that stage for so long without knowing what her glucose level is?* I wondered. *Man,* I thought, *that takes guts.*

"Guess what else?" Paul added. "She wears a pump."

"She wears a pump?" I asked, incredulous. "Where is it? How does she wear a pump in that dress?" She had on a form-fitting, floor-length gown which allowed no room for the lumps, bumps, and tubing that come with a pump.

I read about Miss Johnson in the *Washington Post* while on the subway the next morning. I read about how she was diagnosed at age nineteen. She'd been a young adult, like me, when her life changed forever. I read about how she'd been told she would never have a career or a family. I read that she now wore an insulin pump to treat her diabetes and that she had taken the pump off—she had disconnected the beeper-like device from the tubing—so that it wouldn't show in the evening gown competition. I read that she pricked her finger before the final competition and had a glucose level of 168. Miss Johnson, now Miss America, did not hide her diabetes from the world. She talked about it unashamedly. I thought she might possibly be one of the bravest people I had ever seen.

Speaking of brave, enter, several years later, Supreme Court Justice Sonia Sotomayor. Although Justice Sotomayor is most well known for being the first Hispanic person on the Court, to me and millions of others like me, her significance lies in the fact that she has Type 1 diabetes. Diagnosed as a child, at the age of seven I believe, Justice Sotomayor has talked publicly about her life as a child fifty years ago with Type 1 diabetes. She has described how she ran out of the hospital when, after weeks of unquenchable thirst and bed wetting, she had to have blood drawn and was frightened by the needle; how she saw, for the first time ever, her mother crying when she heard the diagnosis; how she, as a young girl, had to pull a chair over to the stove and boil water to sterilize the needles for her injections of insulin.

Here's another thing that she has said—in my view the most important thing, to the most important audience—the children who have diabetes. She told them they could become anything they wanted to be. The message Miss America had received when she was diagnosed—that she wouldn't be able to have a career or a family—wasn't the message the children who have Type 1 diabetes were getting anymore.

Justice Sotomayor also told the children that she knew it was bad to have diabetes, but it wasn't so bad. Simple words, directed at children, but they struck right at the heart of the matter. Diabetes is bad, but it's not so bad. There are a lot of worse things. And there must be a lot of worse things than wearing an insulin pump. Just look at Miss America.

26

The tubeless pump that Dr. Starr mentioned to me wasn't really what I wanted to hear about. It left me with little reason to continue to resist switching over to pump therapy. My main objections to the pump had always been that I didn't want to have a tube coming out of my body and that I didn't want to have to wear the pump on my body. At least that's what I thought my objections were, yet the news of a cordless pump didn't come as a relief to me. Shouldn't that have been good news if the tube and the pump were really what I was concerned about?

I had to admit to myself that my hesitation wasn't just because of the design of the device. I was terrified to start something new. It had taken me so long to adjust to my life with Type 1 diabetes. It had been the single most difficult thing I'd ever had to face in my life, a life that didn't lack for difficulties. But I had adjusted. Eventually I had adjusted. Now I found myself afraid to start something new yet again. I was afraid of learning a new routine. I was afraid of having a device attached to me that pumped insulin in constantly. I was an insulin-dependent diabetic who was afraid of insulin. I may as well have been a turtle afraid of her own shell.

I took one step forward that day at the doctor's office. I asked Dr. Starr for information about the different types of pumps that were available, including the new tubeless one. I left with the brochures, and I actually read them. I read every word. I looked at every picture. I watched every promotional video. I read every user testimonial. I had to admit at the end of the day, as much as I didn't want to face it, the pump itself didn't seem that scary. It was just that I was scared.

It was I who needed to muster up the nerve to take the plunge and muster the energy to learn a new way of life again.

The brochures remained in a stack on the floor of my bedroom. I noticed them most every day but never paged through them again. I'd think about the pump from time to time, whenever I didn't have a new syringe handy, whenever I had to duck out of a meeting to sneak a shot of insulin, whenever I let my glucose level run too high so I could make it through the many events of my day without worrying about a low.

Those brochures had been on my floor for a full three months when I returned to Dr. Starr for my twelve-week blood work. I told myself that if my A1C was higher than it had been at my last appointment, I would make the leap. As it turned out, my A1C was exactly the same as it had been for my appointment three months earlier. It was higher than it had been the year before and higher than it had been six months before as well, but looking just at a three-month snapshot, it had not gone up. *Phew*, I thought. *I can wait another three months.* It was a silly and dangerous game to play, but I was playing it.

That very night, the night of the day when I'd gotten the results of my blood work, I lay in bed reading a book. One of the characters in the book was a woman whose eyesight was failing. She refused to see an eye doctor because she didn't want to wear glasses. Another character remarked that he couldn't believe she would be so offhand about something as important as her eyesight. What was she waiting for—did she think her eyesight was going to get better?

These were throwaway lines in the book. They weren't central to the plot. They were included only to demonstrate how set in her ways this particular character was. They took up probably eight or ten lines of a book that was a few hundred pages long. In the overall scheme of the book, they were inconsequential. Yet to me, these lines were monumental. *That's what I'm doing*, I thought to myself. *I'm being offhand about my eyes, my heart, my kidneys, all kinds of things.* What was I waiting for? Did I think my diabetes was going to go away? Did I think it was going to get easier to manage? If I had learned one thing during the past many years, it was that my diabetes was here to stay. It wasn't going to get easier to manage. It was always going to be hard.

In that moment, as I contemplated those lines from the book I was reading, I decided I would start on the pump.

The next morning I told Paul, who had been sleeping at the time of my epiphany. "I'm calling Dr. Starr today. I'm going to go on the pump." It took all my courage to tell him, to actually say it out loud.

Paul treated my announcement with none of the gravity it deserved. "That's great, babe. You should do it." He kissed me on the cheek and then was out the door, on his way to work. It's not that he didn't understand how hard this decision was for me. I think it was more likely that he didn't believe me. I'd been talking about the pump for so long yet doing nothing about it, and he probably thought I was just talking again.

Even my young daughter was used to hearing me talk about the pump. One day, when I had my cell phone clipped to my belt, which isn't a look I usually go for but one I had adopted as a matter of necessity that day, she said to me, "Well, I guess you finally did it, Mommy."

"Finally did what?" I asked.

"You finally got the diabetes pump. I see it there on your belt," she responded. She had heard me so many times describe the pump as being about the size of a cell phone, and she had heard me so many times say it has to be attached to your belt. I hated knowing my diabetes had such a central role in her thoughts.

I also hated thinking of myself as someone who talked about taking action but didn't actually act. I'm not usually that sort of person. I'm not a big talker. I'm a doer. I'm careful not to say I'm going to do something unless I *am* going to do it. What Paul hadn't noticed when I made my announcement that morning was that I hadn't used the same words I usually used when I talked about the pump. The words I usually used were equivocal, along the lines of, "I know I'll have to go on the pump one of these days." The words I'd said to Paul were definitive words. I'd made an affirmative statement, aloud, to another human being: "I'm going to go on the pump." This subtle distinction was lost on him. But for me, having said it, there was no turning back.

I called Dr. Starr that day. Ever responsive, he returned my call that same afternoon. I told him that I'd made up my mind. I was going on the pump. I was going to try the new tubeless one that he had told me about several months earlier.

"That's great. I think you'll really be happy with it," he said.

"So what's the next step?" I asked. "Do I need to make an appointment to come in and see you?"

"Oh, no, no. You don't see me for this. I'll give you the name of a pump trainer to call. She'll get you started." *What?* Dr. Starr, the person I had grown to rely on and trust more than anyone else in my complicated medical world, wasn't going to train me on the pump? I heard a dull screeching noise in my head, like brakes being slammed on and a long skid ensuing. I hadn't bargained for this when I had made my announcement. I was reminded of the shock I'd felt on that day seven and a half years ago when I'd learned that the doctor who had seen me through thirty-six weeks of pregnancy wouldn't deliver my baby.

"You don't show me how to use the pump?" I asked, surprised, when I had caught my breath and could speak again.

"No, no. I'll see you once you get regulated. But I don't train you on the technical side of it. There are trainers who do that."

Great, trainers, I thought. *Another new person to add to my team. Another set of appointments.* "They aren't the sales reps, are they?" I knew a little about the medical equipment sales industry, and I didn't want to turn the care of my diabetes over to an equipment sales rep.

"Oh, no. This'll be a nurse—someone who specializes in diabetes care but who's also up to speed on all the pump technology."

"Okay," I said, more loudly than necessary, trying to overcome with volume the quaking in my voice. "How do I get set up with a trainer?"

"There are some forms you need to fill out. Some papers that I'll have to submit to your insurance company to make sure they'll pay for the pump."

"Is there a question as to that?" I asked, alarmed. "Is it possible my insurance won't pay?" The cost of being on an insulin pump is several thousand dollars per year. This is in addition to the cost of the insulin itself and the cost of glucose test strips.

"Remind me how many shots you're taking a day. I don't have your file right here," he said.

"Four or five usually," I told him.

"And what was your last A1C?" he asked.

I told him.

"They'll pay," he said. "I'm sure they'll pay. I'll fill out my part of the forms and fax them over to you. Then you fill out your part and fax them back. Once we hear from your insurance company, I'll put you in touch with the right trainer."

I received the insurance forms from the doctor promptly. I reviewed his answers to the various questions in the physician section of the forms. In response to the question, "How long is patient's condition expected to persist?" he had written in his physician's scrawl, "for the rest of her life." Of course, I knew that was the answer, but it was a kick in the gut to see it in black and white. Sighing wearily, I completed my part of the forms and sent them back to him.

More quickly than I would have liked, my insurance company approved full reimbursement of the cost of my pump. I don't mean to be glib by this statement. I've been exceedingly fortunate during all stages of my disease, including during the all-important time of my pregnancy, to have comprehensive medical insurance coverage. My life and the life of everyone in my family would be very different if I didn't have insurance to cover the vast majority of the many expenses associated with managing Type 1 diabetes. I know this, and I am grateful for it every day of my life.

But I was still scared to start on the pump. I was trying to act brave, trying to fool myself, but it wasn't working. So I'd hoped for a little lag time, a few weeks while I waited to hear from my insurance company. That way, I would've taken a solid first step toward making good on my public announcement that I was going to start on the pump, but if it didn't actually happen for a long time, I could chalk it up to insurance glitches. I had no such luck. There were no insurance glitches. My insurance company approved the pump within days of my forms being submitted.

Dr. Starr called me with the news. "Okay, we got the insurance approval," he said. "So you can order the pump and set up an appointment with your trainer. Did I give you the name of anyone yet?"

"No," I answered. "You said you'd tell me the name of someone once you heard back from the insurance company."

"Right. Well, I have someone whom you're really going to like. Do you have a pen? I'll tell you her name and number."

"Yep, ready," I said, my trembling pen poised to write.

"Her name's Caryn Hope," he said, "and her number is...." His voice trailed off. Had I heard him correctly? Could I believe my ears? I thought I had heard him say the most beautiful name I had ever heard. A lyrical name, a tooth-fairy name. If I had heard tires screeching to a halt days ago when I had learned Dr. Starr wouldn't be my pump trainer, I now heard harps playing and saw clouds parting. *Caryn Hope*, I thought to myself.

"What did you say her name is?" I interrupted him. I must have misheard him.

"Caryn Hope," he repeated. "And here's her cell phone number. Just give her a call, and she will get you set up."

I hung up the phone. *Caryn Hope*. What a name, I marveled still. In a world where bad omens sometimes seem to outnumber the good, I need to look for good omens wherever I can find them. Here, in this woman's name, I believed I'd found one. "Caryn" sounds like caring. Hope, I don't even need to explain that one. Caryn

Hope. I felt good about this. I was so glad he hadn't set me up with an Ida Kilmore.

I talked to Caryn Hope on the phone a few days later. I was not disappointed. She lived up to all my expectations. She personified every characteristic that I'd expected from someone with such a propitious name. She was energetic, enthusiastic, optimistic, knowledgeable, reassuring, calm, and happy. I heard all of these qualities in her voice, in her tone, in her choice of words during our first conversation. If there was anyone who could get me through this transition, she was the one. I could tell. I couldn't wait to meet her. Before I could meet her, however, I had to order the pump. Those were my marching orders from her: order the pump, call her when I received it, and then she'd come to my home and train me on how to use it.

27

The large box remained virtually undisturbed for a while before I worked up the nerve to call Caryn Hope again. After I'd opened the box and reviewed its contents, I packed everything back inside, closed it up, and dragged the box into different rooms of my house in an effort to find a place where it wouldn't distract me. It hadn't left me alone when I left it in the front hall. Nor in my bedroom. Nor under the kitchen table. Nor in my home office. Its presence cast a pall over any room where I put it. The box contained my new insulin pump.

Before the pump arrived I had tried and almost succeeded in fooling myself into believing that I was excited about moving into this new phase of treatment. After all, I had answered in the affirmative and without hesitation all of the questions in the promotional brochure for the pump:

Are you tired of taking up to five injections of insulin a day to control your diabetes? Yes.

Are you fearful of low blood sugar and tired of snacking all the time to deal with it? Yes.

Are you struggling to reach your target blood sugar levels and frustrated with a lifestyle of injection after injection? Yes and yes.

Do you want more flexibility in your day-to-day schedule? Yes.

Yet when the pump arrived, the size of the box in which it was delivered disturbed me. I was expecting a small box, perhaps a size that would hold a cell phone or a calculator. The pump itself—though I had never seen a real, live one—was said to be smaller than a computer mouse. So why was the box that was left sitting on my doorstep big enough to house a mid-sized dog?

I knew the pump was coming. Following Caryn Hope's instructions, I had ordered it. The manufacturer had sent an email to let me know that it had been shipped. *Please, let it be coming from far, far away,* I thought to myself. *Please let it have to traverse mountain passes on the back of a crippled donkey. Please let it have to cross an ocean on a steamer. Please let it take a really long time to get here.* DHL proved to be more reliable than that.

"There's a box at the front door!" Emily squealed as we pulled into the driveway. "What do you think it is? Maybe it's for me!"

I couldn't imagine what it was. I was expecting my insulin pump to be delivered any day, but there was no way that large box at my door was my insulin pump. It was just too big.

"I'm gonna go see who it's for," Emily said, bolting from the car the instant I parked it. I hadn't yet unloaded all of our belongings from the car when Emily ran back, breathless, and announced, "It's for you, Mommy. It says Amy Ryan."

"Did you see who it's from?" I asked.

"I couldn't tell... come on, come on, let's go," she said, pulling my arm and leading me toward the box.

When we got to the box, I confirmed that my name was on the shipping label and then looked at the name on the return address. It was the name of the pump manufacturer. This wasn't making any sense to me. I lugged the box inside, hoisted it onto the dining room table, and let it rest there.

"Well, who's it from? Aren't you going to open it?" Emily asked. The idea of not tearing open a box the instant you lay eyes on it is not comprehensible to a seven-year-old. Only good things are delivered in boxes to a seven-year-old. I had to play this one carefully. Emily could sense my stress ten miles away. I didn't want her to think that the pump was anything other than a good thing. Time to fake nonchalance.

Turning on my carefree voice, my I-will-try-not-to-let-her-know-how-scared-I-am voice, I responded, "I'm not sure, but I think it's that new diabetes thing—the insulin pump I've been talking about."

"Well, aren't you going to open it?"

"Oh, I will. I just want to get dinner started first. I'll open it later. Why don't you go outside and play, and take the dog with you." Obedient as always, she slipped out the back door with the dog.

I didn't really care about getting dinner started. What I really wanted was to get used to the box. And I wanted to be alone when I opened it. If I was disturbed when its contents were revealed to me, if I wanted to wallow in a moment or two of self-pity, if I wanted to swear or to scream or to cry, I didn't want my daughter to be my witness. It's tough enough to have a mom who's been known to lick the blood off her throbbing fingertip when there's not a tissue handy; a mom who exposes her fleshy abdomen and inserts a needle into it so many times a day that we lose count; a mom who says embarrassing things that people sometimes misunderstand. "I need to do a shot," and "I'm so high," have much different meanings outside the world of diabetes. It's tough enough to deal with all of that, so I would at least spare my daughter my reaction when I opened the box.

After shooing Emily out the back door, I poured myself a glass of wine, a very tall glass of wine, found some scissors, and slit open the packing tape around the box. I opened it at the top. Styrofoam macaroni spilled out over the edges. I put my hands into the macaroni and fished around slowly, cautiously, trying to spill as little of it as possible. I came across something solid, a case of some sort. I got my hands around it and pulled it out. It was a stylized leatherette case, sort of like a briefcase, only smaller. More like the size of a notebook, a three-ring binder. I placed it carefully on the dining room table and brushed the residue of the styrofoam packaging materials off its surface. Turning it over, I examined the case tentatively. There was a zipper around three sides of it. I took a deep breath, pulled the zipper around all three sides, and opened it up. On the left side was a user guide. On the right side was the device I'd been expecting, the cellphone sized computer device. There was also one pod. The pod was the tubeless device I would fill with insulin and attach to my body.

I was relieved to see the size of the pod, the thing I'd actually be wearing. It really didn't seem that big. It was about the shape of a computer mouse and about two-thirds the size. At a glance, it seemed like something I could hide under my clothes pretty easily.

The computer device, my new "PDM"—which stands for personal diabetes manager—was something else altogether. It looked to me to be very complicated, judging by the buttons on it. This device would now be my glucose monitor, the machine into which I would insert a test strip whenever I pricked my finger. It would also control, through a wireless communication system, the continuous delivery of insulin from the pod on my body through the cannula, or tube, that would be under my skin. Whereas my current glucose meter had only two keys, this new device had ten keys on it. There were three unlabeled keys situated horizontally beneath the display screen. Below those were up and down arrow keys, similar to scrolling keys on a keyboard, centered over a square key with a graphic depiction of a light bulb on it. There was a key with a house graphic on it, a key with a knife and fork on it, a key with a question mark on it, and a key with the all-familiar, teardrop-shaped drop of blood on it.

I'm a technophobe. I don't Tweet. I don't have a Facebook page. I don't know how to use an iPod. I've never downloaded a song or a video. I can send a text message only under the close supervision of a teenager. I found the look of my new PDM to be incredibly intimidating. *The kids will think it's cool*, I thought to myself, but that's about as positive a feeling as I had. Hoping to be reassured that I would in fact be able to operate this little gadget, I pried the user manual out of the case. No, wait, let me make one clarification: I pried the 159-page user manual out of the case. I sighed and shook my head as I thumbed through the manual. This could not be easy to learn if it required 159 pages to explain it.

I felt a feeling that I hadn't experienced in a long time, one that I hadn't missed at all, creeping up on me. I started to feel heavy, literally dragged down. I felt as if I were moving through molasses.

Maybe I wasn't ready for this. I certainly didn't feel like I had the energy for it just then. I returned the manual to its case and zipped the case closed, trusting in the principle that what I couldn't see wouldn't scare me.

So now I had seen what accounted for a small percentage of the size of the box—what else could be inside? I eased my hands back into the box and fished around until I felt something else solid. I scraped the macaroni aside. I saw what took up the rest of the volume of the box: new supplies. There were several boxes of replacement pods—each pod full of insulin has to be removed, discarded and replaced every three days—alcohol pads with a mild adhesive solution, and adhesive removal cream. The moment I saw all of these supplies, I felt stupid, naïve. Why I hadn't I guessed this? How could I not have realized that with a new treatment regime would come a whole new set of supplies? My mind raced back to that night over a decade before, when I'd sat alone in my apartment, trying to figure out my new glucose meter, not understanding that the ten test strips that came with the new machine would not get me through three days. Was it going to be that bad again? Was the learning curve going to be as steep as it had been then, the anxiety and adjustment processes as painful?

As I stood gazing at my new collection of supplies, Emily ran back into the house through the back door. "So you opened it," she exclaimed, breathless from running around outside.

"I did, yes, I sure did," was my noncommittal answer.

"Well, how do you like it?" she persisted.

"Like it?" I asked, still distracted. I caught myself and snapped out of it. "Oh, I *love* it," I said, smiling and feigning enthusiasm. Then, just to set the stage for what I was concerned might be a difficult transition for me, I added, "It's going to be a lot to learn. But once I figure it out, I think it'll be awesome." She looked at me and smiled, relieved. She was tired of worrying about my diabetes, too.

I once told Emily, when she was nervous about giving a presentation in front of her class, that she should pretend to be brave. Just fake it. Pretend that you're brave, and everyone will think you are. They won't know what you're thinking inside. Before you know it, you'll forget that you were pretending, and you'll find out that you really are brave. I was pretending to be brave with her. I was hoping the real thing would kick in soon. Caryn Hope would have her work cut out for her.

When I finally called her to say my pump had arrived, "That's terrific!" was her enthusiastic response. As I spent more time with her, I would learn that Caryn Hope thought most things were terrific. If you told her you have diabetes, she'd be likely to say, "You do? You're so lucky—this is a terrific time to have diabetes," and then she'd go on to tell you all the great things about life for people with diabetes in the 21st century. And the amazing thing is, you'd believe her. You'd come away from your encounter with her, scratching your head and thinking in spite of yourself, *Wow, she's right. I am lucky.* Her optimism was contagious. If they could bottle that, I would happily inject it every day.

Caryn told me to pick a week when I didn't have a lot going on, a week that would be relatively stress-free, for me to be trained and regulated on the pump. I should start on a Monday. On the Thursday or Friday before that Monday, she would come over and get me going on a dummy pump, a pump filled with saline rather than insulin, so I could practice wearing it and operating it before going live.

"A week?" I asked. "Is it going to take a whole week for me to figure this out?"

"We'll have to see. Everybody's different," Caryn began in her typically calming fashion. "Some people are regulated within a few days; other people may take a few weeks. We'll see how it goes. I'm guessing you'll have it figured out pretty quickly." It seemed like she always finished on a high note.

We ended the conversation with my promise to check my calendar for a week that looked clear for the training. A light week is not something that comes along very often in my calendar. I remembered her comment that it could take a few weeks for me to get regulated on the pump. I was more encouraged than disheartened by that comment. Perhaps it would take a few weeks for me to learn my new routine on the pump. Perhaps she would tell me I needed to take a few weeks off work, or maybe she would say that I should spend lots of time at the pool during those weeks, just to be sure the pump operates in the sweltering heat and when soaked with chlorinated pool water. Perhaps she'd say that during those few weeks, I shouldn't do laundry or cook dinner or do anything else I didn't want to do. Or she'd tell me to read lots of books, enjoy long, soaking baths, and generally pamper myself. I was deep into this daydream when I decided to call Caryn for a reality check.

"No, a week off work should do it," she said. "I wouldn't think you'd need to take more time than that." So, okay, there'd be no rest for the weary. I was pretty much going to have to make this change and keep trudging ahead with business and life as usual. The world wasn't going to wait for me to adjust to the new challenges of my daily life. It wasn't even going to slow down a little. Paul and the kids were going to keep needing me, my work at the office was going to keep piling up, and I was going to have to buck up once again and learn to live my new life. Not even Caryn Hope could stop the world from spinning.

I hadn't told a lot of people at work about my diabetes. My secretary knew, and she kept my medical information in a manual at her desk in case she ever needed to summon emergency help for me. A handful of other friends at work knew—mostly the few people with whom I socialized outside of work, where I felt I could be a little more open about my condition. But for the most part, I'd hidden my condition from most of my colleagues at work for a long time, nearly eight years.

Perhaps hidden isn't the right word. It wasn't an intentional act of hiding. It was just continuing passive omission. There never seemed to be a good time to bring it up. It was like when a new neighbor moves in next door, and you don't introduce yourself at first. You mean to stop by, knock on the door, and welcome her, but then somehow you never find the time. The longer you take to make your introduction, the more awkward it becomes, until finally you never introduce yourself, and you never even meet that neighbor.

I had approached my diabetes much the same way. I'd never found the right time to bring it up, and so in many cases I never had. There was one time in my career, early on, that I had mentioned it to a colleague. I was going to his office for a conference call with a client. Before leaving my office for his, I pricked my finger to get a glucose reading, as I always did before I left my office for any period of time. I got my result and knew I was headed for a low. I wasn't low yet—I was fine at that moment—but I knew from my glucose level that if I didn't get some glucose into me in the next half hour, I was in for a crash. That isn't the best news to get on your way to a meeting. I gobbled down a few glucose pills, tucked my glucose meter into the expandable file that I was carrying, and headed down to his office. I knew I'd need to prick my finger again in about fifteen minutes to be sure my glucose level was headed in the right direction, which in this case would be up.

I had pricked my finger surreptitiously in this person's office before. It was generally easy to do. We usually sat at a table together when we worked. He would excuse himself from time to time to walk back over to his desk to check his e-mail, or to step out for a moment to get some water or tea, which he was kind enough always to offer me as well. I would take these little opportunities to hide my glucose meter under the table and do a quick test. On this occasion, however, I wouldn't be able to hide my testing from him. I'd need to prick my finger just a few minutes after our conference call started, so I couldn't wait until he had stepped away for a moment. There was no getting around it.

Before the start of the call, I swallowed hard and then broke the news to him. I told him I had diabetes, that my glucose level was getting a little low, and I'd need to prick my finger to get a glucose reading several minutes into the call. I told him there wasn't any cause for alarm. I just might need to eat something during the call. I wanted to let him know what I'd be doing and why I might be chomping on glucose pills.

He accepted the news graciously, and we proceeded with the call. About ten minutes into it, I pricked my finger: 158. Phew. The glucose pills I'd taken before I had left my office had worked their magic. Although 158 is too high for the average nondiabetic person, for an insulin-dependent diabetic trying to get through a long conference call, 158 is a sight for sore eyes. My colleague had seen me prick my finger and do the glucose test. He had watched curiously, as anyone might. When I had packed up my kit and put it away, he muted the phone and asked in a hushed tone, "Is everything okay?"

I smiled and gave him the thumbs up. "I'm in good shape," I whispered back. He smiled back, relieved. He unmuted the phone, and we continued with our call.

After the call was over, he asked me a few of the usual questions about my condition. I answered forthrightly, if a bit briefly. No, I can't control my diabetes with diet and exercise. Yes, I have to take insulin. No, I'm not part of the epidemic. Yes, four shots on a good day. Actually, that's in addition to the finger pricks. Probably about ten or twelve of those a day. Yes, that's what Julia Roberts had in *Steel Magnolias*. Yes, being pregnant had been a challenge. No, there's not a cure.

He shook his head in disbelief. "Wow, that sounds like a lot to deal with," he said.

"At times, it really is," I said. "But you get used to it, you know? It just becomes routine." I try to make people feel at ease about my condition. I don't want anyone to worry about me.

This guy, however, did worry about me. From that day on, whenever I was in his office for a meeting, which was several times a week, he'd ask me, "Is your blood sugar okay? Do you need to do a test on your blood? Just let me know if you need to eat or take a break."

He was trying, sincerely, to be nice. He was trying to let me know that he was aware of my health needs and didn't want our work to get in the way of my need to monitor my glucose levels and treat my diabetes. Despite his good motives, I was very uncomfortable whenever he made these comments. They said to me that the first thing this guy thought about every time he saw me was my diabetes. I didn't want diabetes to define me. I didn't want people to see me and think, *There's that diabetic woman.* I didn't want to be labeled.

After this had happened several times, I decided I had to say something to him about it. I told him I appreciated his concern, which I honestly did, but I'd rather that he not ask me about my diabetes every time we met. I let him know that I'd certainly tell him if I anticipated running into any problems during a meeting with him, and that I'd feel comfortable pulling out my meter and checking my glucose level in his company whenever I needed to, but beyond that he should assume that I had things under control. He seemed relieved and slightly embarrassed to hear this. He had been worried about me, and he hadn't known what to do with that worry. "I'm really fine," I assured him. "You don't need to worry."

That experience confirmed that I'd been right to be cautious about revealing my big secret. Now that I was about to take a week of medical leave to get regulated on my new pump, I had to decide how much I should tell my co-workers about why I was taking the leave. I wanted it to be known that this was medical leave. It was mid-June, and people might logically assume that a week out of the office was a week of vacation. The problem was, I was taking a real vacation in August. When the time for my real vacation rolled around, about six weeks later, I didn't want people to say, "Weren't you just on vacation?" The week I would spend getting trained on the pump would be anything but vacation.

"Medical leave? Is everything okay?" each of my co-workers asked, genuinely concerned. A woman taking medical leave is an enigma to her co-workers. People are not sure what they can ask. Some might assume that she must have had a miscarriage or a hysterectomy or some other "female" problem. Others worry that it might be breast cancer. Still others might assume cosmetic surgery. I was concerned that the speculation about my mysterious leave might lead people to believe I was facing a situation more dire than it actually was.

I decided to tell people why I'd be out of the office. I decided to finally tell them I had Type 1 diabetes and I would be starting on an insulin pump to try to get better control of my disease. I needed the time out of the office to get trained on the pump and to get my glucose levels regulated. The first time I said it out loud, the first time I heard myself explaining to a colleague on the phone why I'd be out of the office, my voice wavered and cracked. Actually, I was still terrified of switching over to the pump. The more people I told, the more real it became, and that was frightening.

But it wasn't just that. I felt sorry for myself—not in a self-pitying sort of way—but in the way of a sympathetic outsider, looking in at everything I had dealt with and thinking, *That poor woman, it's not enough that she has to do this thing that frightens her so, she also has to tell these private details of her life to her co-workers.*

To a person, everyone I told about my transition to the pump was extremely supportive—so supportive, in fact, that I probably could've taken the summer off to lounge by the pool, and no one would have blinked an eye. They really just wanted to know that I was going to be all right. Many were shocked to learn that I had diabetes, or they wondered whether this meant my diabetes was getting worse, and some even thought it meant I was having a pancreas transplant or a medical device surgically implanted. A few asked the question that's so hard to hear, the one I hated to answer the most: "An insulin pump—will that cure your diabetes?"

28

A few years earlier, when Emily was still a baby, Willie met me at my car one evening when I got home from work. As soon as he saw my car round the corner, he ran out of the house toward me, waving a slip of paper in his hand. *What now?* I thought to myself. If someone was running out to meet me, it could only mean calamity: The boys had been fighting, or the dog had soiled the carpet, or the washing machine had overflowed.

But on that day, Willie was excited. He had run out to greet me with some happy news.

Catching his breath after his dash to the car, he announced, "The American Diabetes Association called. I told them you'd be home at 7:00. They said you can call them back. Here's their phone number." He handed me the slip of paper as I got out of the car.

"Thanks, Willie," I responded offhandedly as I opened the back door of the car, disengaged Emily's car seat, and heaved it out to carry her into the house. *What a good boy,* I thought to myself. He'd actually written down a phone number and given me a message. That was a first.

I went into the house and began my daily unloading ritual. I gently put down the sleeping baby, still in her car seat, in the corner of the kitchen. I unloaded the diaper bag, put the empty bottles in the sink, and started to organize for dinner.

"Amy, it's almost 7:15," Willie said impatiently. He'd been following me around the kitchen, waiting for me to pick up the phone and return the message. "I told the diabetes people you'd be home around 7:00. You need to call them back."

"I'm not going to call them back, sweetie," I said, not missing a beat as I continued to rummage around the kitchen.

"But why not?" Willie asked, visibly stricken by my response.

"Because they're probably just calling to see if I want to renew my magazine subscription, and I don't want to right now."

"But what if that's not why they're calling? What if they're calling to tell you there's a cure?"

I froze in my tracks. My breath caught in my throat. A cure. Willie thought there was a cure. And he thought he was the one who had delivered the message to me.

Delicately, I said, "Willie, honey, there's not a cure. That's not why they're calling."

"But how do you know? What if there's a cure, and you just don't know about it?"

"Well," I paused as if to consider the question. I then did my best to formulate a response that might make sense to an eight-year-old. "I think if there was a cure I'd hear about it on the news. Or I'd read about it in my diabetes magazine. And my doctor would definitely call me if there was a cure."

"But still..." He was disappointed by my cynicism. He didn't want to let this go so easily.

Facing him, I put my hands gently on his shoulders and looked down into his doleful eyes. I studied his fresh, hopeful face. "You're right," I said, as if I'd reconsidered and now saw some merit in his point. "I should call them back. You never know." He sprang up on his toes, his mood lifted by my faith in his theory, in his belief there might be a cure. "Let me go upstairs and change out of my work clothes, and I'll call them from up there."

I'd just employed one of my key mechanisms for coping in front of the kids, maybe one of my key mechanisms for coping in general: I'd faked it. I'd faked belief in Willie's theory about a cure. I would fake the phone call to the diabetes association. When I recounted for Willie the results of the imaginary call, I'd fake indifference that there is not, in fact, a cure. I'd conclude by shrugging in a carefree manner and giving him a fake report that a cure is probably just around the corner.

I was still new to the disease when I realized for the first time that a cure might not be just around the corner. The day I was told I had to start taking insulin, my endocrinologist told me not to despair, that a cure was five years off, ten years at the outside. *I can do this for five years, maybe even ten if I have to,* I had thought at the time.

Around the same time, I read a letter to the editor in a diabetes-focused magazine. A frustrated person with Type I diabetes had written to the editor to lament that no cure for diabetes had been found: "Twenty years ago, my doctor told me we could count on a cure in the next twenty years. Last month I read that a cure may be ten to twenty years away. Will I be reading this same thing in another ten years—that a cure is probably just ten years away?" I read his letter over and over. The weight of his words settled over me. *There's not going to be a cure in ten years,* I realized.

A cure is not something I let myself think about. It's not something I can even conceptualize. I can scarcely recall what life was like before I had diabetes. I don't remember not knowing what a glucose level is. I don't remember smooth fingertips whose only insult was an occasional splinter. I don't remember the skin on my abdomen and thighs not being marred by contusions and sore spots from endless injections of insulin. I don't remember falling asleep at night without wondering whether my glucose level was high enough to get me through the night. I don't remember leaving the house with only car keys in hand, without the many supplies that are needed to keep me going. I don't remember having my foot fall asleep and not being stricken with gut-wrenching terror that I'm losing the feeling in that foot. I don't remember waking up bleary-eyed without wondering whether the blurry vision is because I haven't yet shaken my sleep or because my eyesight is finally starting to go.

Although there isn't a cure, new technologies for the treatment of diabetes have been developed just during my lifetime with the disease. On the glucose-testing front, there's a technology that promises to make finger pricking a thing of the past. The continuous glucose monitor, or CGM, monitors glucose levels on a nearly continuous basis through a sensor device that is worn on the body. The device that's attached to the skin is smaller than the insulin pod that I'd soon be wearing. It's more like the size of a square Band-Aid and nearly as slim. A sensor inserted under the skin reads the glucose level and wirelessly transmits the result every few seconds to a handheld radio receiver. It can predict trends in glucose levels, upward or downward, and it signals an alarm when the glucose level is rising or falling too quickly.

The CGM has the potential to give newfound freedom to people like me who test their glucose levels a dozen times a day. This freedom could let us go for a jog, take a nap, run errands, go to a movie, go for a drive, with a real-time report of what our glucose level is doing. The CGM can take a lot of the fear and guesswork out of the daily challenges of managing life on insulin.

With all the benefits the CGM offers, there are, of course, a few drawbacks. The sensor doesn't measure the glucose level in the blood, because the sensor isn't inserted intravenously. Rather, it measures the glucose level in the fluid that surrounds the cells in our bodies, also known as interstitial fluid. The glucose level of interstitial fluid lags behind the glucose level in the blood. Although a lag may not be significant during periods when the glucose level is stable, if it is rising or falling rapidly, a lag could be dangerous if the reported level is not accurate. So finger pricks are still recommended to compare the blood glucose level with the interstitial fluid glucose level.

Finger pricks are also recommended several times a day to calibrate the interstitial fluid glucose levels against the glucose level in the blood. So we're not quite at the point when we can put away our lancing devices, but perhaps we're getting there.

Also on the technology front is an exciting initiative known as the Artificial Pancreas Project. Funded in large part by the Juvenile

Diabetes Research Foundation, the Artificial Pancreas Project aims to integrate two technologies—the insulin pump and the CGM—into one automatically self-adjusting insulin delivery and glucose monitoring system. The idea behind the artificial pancreas is that the CGM will transmit glucose levels on a real-time basis to an insulin pump, and the insulin pump will adjust automatically the delivery of insulin, based on the then-current glucose level. The amount of insulin to be delivered will be calculated by an algorithm that takes into account many variables that affect the rate at which the body absorbs insulin: what the user will be eating, whether she will be exercising, whether she will be sleeping, and numerous other factors.

These technologies give us hope. They make it easier to manage our disease. They make it easier to get through the day and to sleep through the night. They make it safer to live life on insulin. A cure, though? What about a cure?

I've had friends call me excitedly to tell me they'd read in the paper about a cure for diabetes. Well, actually, they hadn't read the whole article, but they'd seen the headline: "Gene Therapy Reverses Type 1 Diabetes," "Antibodies Reverse Type 1 Diabetes," "Researchers Find Cure for Type 1 Diabetes." Had they read just slightly more than the headline—if they'd read even the first sentence—they'd have seen the two words that don't allow me to let down my guard and believe there might be a cure. Those two words are: "in mice." There are several apparent cures for diabetes in mice. In most of these articles, there are a few other words, too, that I've heard before—five to ten years. More research in mice, clinical trials in humans, but we should be there in five to ten years. That seems to be the magic time frame that we're promised every couple of years.

We're holding on. We're here. We're waiting. What else is there to do? For now, I'd go with the insulin pump.

29

I met Caryn Hope at my home on a Thursday morning. She arrived right on time, as I should've known she would. We walked through my house to the family room, and she couldn't help but notice the state of my dining room and kitchen. There were a mess of cookbooks, casserole dishes, trays, plates, and glasses. There were streamers, a poster-sized collage, and a crumpled up "Congratulations Graduate" banner. My stepson, Ned, the one who had slugged his brother in the arm at the suggestion so many years ago that I might have *die*-betes, was graduating from high school in two days. We were hosting a graduation party the next night.

"My goodness, it looks like you're in the middle of something," Caryn said.

"We're hosting a little party tomorrow night. My stepson graduates from high school on Saturday," I explained.

"I thought you were going to pick a light week to start on the pump," she teased .

"Next week will be light," I assured her. "This weekend will be crazy, but next week will be pretty quiet." The next week, Monday, was when I would actually start on the pump. Today's meeting was for me to get some basic training on how to operate this new device. I would also, at the end of today's meeting, start wearing a dummy pump filled with saline.

We sat down together on the couch in my family room. Caryn reached into her giant tote bag. It reminded me of Mary Poppins' bag, containing all sorts of magic and tricks. She pulled out a file folder containing a few sheets of loose-leaf paper.

"Okay, let's get started," she began. "First, I have this little quiz for you to take, just to be sure you've brushed up on all the basics."

I was good at quizzes. I'd be happy to take a quiz about diabetes. Correction—I'd be happy to *ace* a quiz about diabetes. I must have learned it all by this point. I breezed through the first few questions. And then I stumbled, more than a few times. Turns out I had gotten sloppy with some of my diabetes care. "You did really well!" she said, beaming at me after she read over my answers, marking several as incorrect. Apparently, even screwing up a quiz was great news for Caryn Hope.

After we'd gone over the quiz and Caryn had explained the questions I'd missed, she pulled a few more papers out of her magic bag. She walked me through the basic principles of the insulin pump I'd be wearing. She explained that it was a pod-like device that would be filled with insulin and attached to my body at all times. Each pod would last three days, and then I would take it off, refill another one with insulin, and start again. Each time I put a pod on my body, I would program my PDM—my personal diabetes manager—to insert a needle and cannula under my skin. The needle would retract once the cannula had been inserted, but the cannula, the flexible tubing, would remain under my skin. I would receive a measured, constant dose—the "basal" dose—of fast-acting insulin through the cannula around the clock, and I would program the PDM to release an additional dose of insulin—the "bolus" dose—before each meal and at any other times when my glucose level was too high. Those were the basics.

She explained the benefits of pump therapy, which I'd heard before but loved hearing again: better blood sugar control with fewer episodes of hypoglycemia, meaning fewer lows; less risk of long-term complications from diabetes; flexibility with meal and exercise timing; no more injections once the cannula was inserted every third day.

Then she explained something I hadn't thought much about before: the risks of pump therapy. I hadn't thought of those. Nothing good comes without some risk.

As Caryn explained, the most significant risk of using an insulin pump was that the flow of insulin could be interrupted. I might not know about the interruption, and before too long I could be heading toward diabetic ketoacidosis, or DKA. DKA is the opposite of a low. DKA comes from being way too high. It can come on quickly. It's the condition that I had when I was initially diagnosed so many years ago. DKA can lead to coma and, if not caught in time, death.

Before I was on the pump, there was little risk of DKA because I always had a base level of insulin from the long-acting dose that I gave myself every twenty-four hours. Once I switched over to the pump, however, I'd no longer be taking long-acting insulin. I'd only be receiving the short-acting insulin delivered through the cannula. If the cannula became clogged or dislodged, or if there was any other interruption in the delivery of insulin, I'd only have a few hours' worth of a low dose of short-acting insulin in my system. This meant I'd be only a few hours away from DKA if my insulin delivery were interrupted and I didn't remedy it quickly.

"If that were to happen, if my pump malfunctioned and I wasn't getting any insulin, how long would it take before I ran into real trouble? Would it be hours? Days?"

"Definitely not days," Caryn responded, her tone serious. "Hours. You could be seriously ill within hours."

"How many hours?"

"Well, I can't give you an exact number, but probably eight to ten."

I tried to keep breathing calmly while I considered that new information. I was used to being worried about lows. Lows are the constant vexation of every person who uses insulin. I didn't like worrying about lows, but at least I was used to that. I was not used to being worried on a daily basis about highs. Granted, highs are not good. Highs will eventually lead to long-term complications. But on a daily basis, highs weren't a threat. They had to be dealt with, they had to be treated with insulin, but it wasn't likely they'd be my immediate demise because of the long-acting insulin in my system.

Slowing down only briefly to let me absorb this information, Caryn showed me how to program my PDM. She used a worksheet to calculate what my initial basal rate of insulin would be, and she entered that number into the PDM. She used another worksheet to calculate how much insulin I should get from a bolus, both to correct a high glucose level before I ate as well as to cover the carbs from what I would eat. She put those calculations into the PDM as well.

"You've got it, right?" she asked, smiling. She could tell that she had lost me somewhere along the line. It all sounded so complicated.

"I'm never going to get this," I moaned.

"You will. The PDM does it all for you. All you have to do is enter your carbs."

"What if I don't remember everything you just explained to me?"

"Amy," she said in as firm a voice as she could muster, "you're going to get this. I've trained a four-year-old on this pump. I have a man who's ninety years old on one of these. He doesn't even know how to use a cell phone, and he figured this out. Believe me, you're going to get it."

Next we filled a pod because with saline—because this was a trial run—using the large syringe that came with it. We synchronized the pod with the PDM so they could communicate with each other, and then the moment of truth arrived: "Prepare infusion site," the display screen on the PDM instructed. That meant the spot on my body where I would wear the pod.

"We're going to start you with a pod on your abdomen. After a month or so, you can start wearing it on your thigh or upper arm, but we like to start on your abdomen because the insulin absorption is more regular there," Caryn explained.

She added that I would need to change the pod every three days. I'd need to put each new pod at least an inch away from where the old one was.

"Let's get a look at your tummy," she said.

I rolled up my shirt and pulled down the waist of my shorts, letting Caryn get a better look. "Now you don't want to get too close to your belly button, and you don't want to get too close to any scars—that can interfere with the absorption," she said, noticing first the scar from my Caesarean section and then one from an appendectomy performed when I was a teenager. She studied the landscape of my abdomen for just a moment. "So I think we should start around here," she said, indicating a site on the right side of my abdomen. "And you can put your next one here," she said, indicating a spot about an inch closer to my middle, "and the one after that could go here," indicating another spot an inch more inside. "Once you've used those three sites, you can move down an inch and repeat the same thing. Then you can move to the left side and do the same thing. So that's..." She paused to calculate the number of sites she had just plotted. "That's twelve sites. That should get you through thirty-six days. Let's shoot for that."

The screen of my PDM was still telling me to prepare my infusion site. Caryn told me to use one of the alcohol pads to clean the site.

"Wipe it really well," She said.

I swabbed the site until it was glistening. Instinctively, I puckered up and prepared to blow on my wet skin to dry it.

"Oh no, don't blow on it," Caryn warned. "You don't want to blow any germs onto that spot. It has to be sterile. Just let it dry naturally. It won't take long."

After my skin was dry, I removed the adhesive backing and placed the pod on my abdomen, being careful to smooth around all the edges of the adhesive and test to see if it was secure.

"Is it on?" I asked, not sure if I had done it the right way.

Caryn checked the adhesive the whole way around the pod. "It's on," she announced. "Great job."

The next step was to hit the key on my PDM that would tell the pod to release the needle and insert the tube under my skin. This was it. "Is it going to hurt?" I asked. Even as I heard myself say that, I thought, *What a silly question. You've pricked your finger more than 30,000 times and given yourself more than 15,000 injections of insulin, and you're worried this is going to hurt?*

"Is it going to hurt?" she repeated, laughing. "Come on, you stick needles in yourself five times a day—you know what it'll feel like."

Translation: Of course it's going to hurt. But it'll be over before you know it, the sting will fade away, and you'll forget all about it until next time. I pressed the start button. I heard a trigger release at about the same time as I felt a sharp sting. The needle had pierced my skin and retracted. The sting faded before I even had time to comment on it. The screen on my PDM announced that the cannula had been inserted and my basal dose was being delivered.

"So I'm hooked up?" I asked Caryn.

She leaned down until she was eye-level with my belly. She craned her head and peered through a tiny viewing window at one end of the pod. Through the window she could see the clear tube properly implanted in my skin. "You're hooked up. You're good."

*   *   *

The first three days, the practice days, all I had to do was get used to what it felt like to wear the pod and practice programming my boluses into the PDM. At first I noticed the pod on my belly much more often than I would've liked. When I was driving in the car, my seatbelt came across my midsection and pressed down right where the pod was. The pod clunked against the kitchen counter while I was making a salad for the graduation party. When Emily came home from school and I hugged her, hoisting her up onto my hip, her weight fell uncomfortably against the pod. When I pulled down my shorts and underpants to use the bathroom, I had to be careful not to accidentally dislodge the pod. But I was not discouraged. With minor changes in my positioning, all of these situations could be dealt with.

One big test was to see what it would feel like to sleep while wearing the pod. I treasured the precious few hours that I spent in bed each night. Paul slept on my left side, and we often held each other tight all through the night. Emily usually ended up on my right side at some point before the sun rose. I didn't want my pod to interfere with our cuddling time.

To my pleasant surprise, the pod was nearly undetectable when I slept. I could sleep on my side, close up against Paul, and feel pretty normal. He just had to get used to an incongruous, plastic bump. I could lie on my stomach, with my full weight bearing down on the pod, and barely notice that it was there. I could roll over onto my right side in the morning and wrap my arms around Emily, just like before.

Paul and I put the pod to the ultimate test on day two. With my clothes off, I was very self-conscious about having it there on my abdomen. It was a glaring imperfection on an already imperfect body. At forty years old, being naked and visible was not as much fun as it used to be, and with a plastic pod stuck on me, the fun factor dipped even farther. From a purely mechanical standpoint, though, the pod didn't interfere with the proceedings. It was there, for sure, but it didn't really get in the way. I didn't have to take it off. I didn't have to worry about it. I didn't have to put my pajamas back on afterward. The tubeless aspect of this type of pump addressed the many concerns I'd had. This was not going to wreck our sex life or even change it that much.

The day of Ned's graduation was the day that my first pod was set to expire. An alarm would sound to remind me that it needed to be changed. I didn't want it to go off during the graduation ceremony, but I didn't know how to prevent that from happening. I called Caryn at 7:30 a.m. to ask her what to do.

I heard a groggy hello, apologized, and asked my question. "Just take it off now, before you go," she said.

I was confused until I remembered it wasn't delivering insulin yet.

"Yep, take it off and deactivate it with your PDM. It's under 'settings' on the main menu. I'll see you on Monday morning for the real thing. And Amy?" Caryn said as I was about to hang up the phone.

"Yes?"

"Congratulations. Enjoy your stepson's graduation." God bless her—she had brought me back to the day.

I hung up the phone, walked into my bathroom, and peeled the pod off my abdomen. I tossed it into the wastebasket. I stared at it for a few seconds and thought, *That's the last time I'll nonchalantly peel off a pod and toss it into the trash. In forty-eight hours that pod will be my lifeline.*

I shivered. Life as I knew it was about to change, again. *Forget about it for now*, I reminded myself. *Enjoy the day.*

30

Caryn came to my house the following Monday. We sat at my dining room table, all my new supplies piled around me.

"So you're ready for this?" she asked, smiling as usual.

I didn't feel ready. I felt paralyzed with fear. "I don't know if I'm ready," I whined. "I don't know why, but I'm just so scared." Then, before I knew it, I was crying. She was sympathetic as I blubbered on, embarrassed about losing control in front of her.

"I'm afraid I'll get too much insulin, and I won't know it," I told her. "I'm afraid I'll have a bad low. I'm afraid the tube will get clogged, and I won't be getting any insulin, and then I'll go into a coma. I'm afraid I'm not going to know what to do."

"You already know what to do," she said. "You learned it last week. We'll go over it again this morning after we get your pod on. And you'll be talking to me every day. A week from now, I'll bet you'll have it mastered."

How I might feel a week from then didn't do much for me at that moment. "Fine. Let's just do it," I said, resigned.

"Okay, get your—"

"No, wait," I interrupted her. "Don't tell me. I want to see if I can do it by following the instructions in the manual." I wanted to make sure I'd know what to do when I needed to change my pod in three days and Caryn wasn't sitting next to me.

Following the instructions, I filled a pod with insulin. I prepped the spot on my abdomen where I would put it. I let the spot dry naturally—I didn't blow on it. I snapped off the needle cap and removed the adhesive backing from the pod. I placed the pod on my lower abdomen. I went through each step slowly, deliberately, raising my eyebrows and looking up for reassurance from Caryn whenever I moved on to the next step. Finally I pushed the button on my PDM to insert the cannula under my skin. I felt the sharp sting—the needle had placed the cannula. The PDM screen told me that the basal dose of insulin was being delivered.

"You're good," Caryn Hope exclaimed.

"I wish I felt good," I said.

"Amy, listen," she said firmly in a tone I hadn't heard before. "You're going to be fine. You know what to do."

She instructed me to call her at home or on her cell phone at 5:00 p.m. to let her know my glucose levels. Then she stood up.

"You're leaving?" I asked, sounding more desperate than I would have liked. I was going to be alone again. Alone to cope. Alone to face the constant vexation, just as I had so many years ago. No one, not even Caryn Hope, could save me from being alone with my disease. *Here I go again*, I thought.

"Call me any time. Call me before five if you need to. But you know what to do. You've got to believe that. You really do know."

"If you say so," I said.

I was alone with the pod. I sat down on the couch and stared at the wall. *What should I do?* Uncharacteristically, I didn't have anything planned. Paul was at work. Emily was at school. Ned, newly graduated and suddenly independent, was at the beach. Willie was asleep in his bedroom downstairs. I had cleared my calendar for my pump training. So what was there for me to do during the hours between finger pricks, meals, and boluses? As if in answer to my question, the phone rang.

It was Spratley.

"Hey—what's going on? I called your office, and your secretary told me you're out on medical leave."

I hadn't talked to her in ages. She had moved away, well out of pajama-walking range, years before.

"Oh, Sprat," I moaned. "I'm not doing so well." Then I quickly clarified, "I mean nothing's wrong—everything's fine. It's just—"

"It's just what?" she broke in. "Why are you on leave?"

"I just started on an insulin pump this morning. A half hour ago, actually," I explained. "I took the week off work so I could get trained on the pump and get my glucose levels regulated. And I'm just all freaked out about it."

"Why do I always show up when you have some diabetes crisis in your life?" she asked.

"Hey, you called me," I replied. "You walked right into this one."

She laughed and said, "Oh, you're going to love it. Just wait and see. One of my son's friends wears an insulin pump, and it's great. His parents say it's changed their lives. And he's nine. Christ, if a nine-year-old can figure it out, you certainly can."

We talked for a few more minutes. I even managed a few laughs. Then I was alone again. I hung up the phone and slumped back into the couch. Then I forced myself up and went through the motions of my daily life. I cleaned up the breakfast dishes. I put in a load of laundry. I made a list of thank-you notes that Ned needed to write for graduation gifts. I found lots of little tasks to fill my morning.

It occurred to me that I would have to get used to life as a "pumper." In addition to my daily finger sticks, I'd have to test my glucose level before I went to sleep at 11:00 p.m. and set my alarm for 1 a.m., so I could wake up, stumble into the bathroom, prick my finger, squint against the light as I wait for the result, and struggle to read it on the screen of the PDM. Then I'd repeat the process at 3:00 a.m., and again at 6:00.

Yet for all I had to do during those first days on the pump, for all the carb counting, record keeping, fine tuning, and sleep deprivation, there was one thing I didn't have to deal with: syringes. In the three days that the pod would be on, I would be spared fifteen shots.

*   *   *

Finally the first three days passed, and it was time for my first pod change without Caryn. I was nervous, of course, but I thought I could do it. Counting the dummy pod full of saline that I wore during the practice period, this would be the third time I'd activated a pod, and I felt like I had the hang of it. Following the instructions to the letter, I executed my first solo pod change without a hitch.

After staying close to home for three days, I decided to venture out into the world. I was going on a bona fide shopping trip. Since I needed to start carrying more supplies with me than I before, I figured I was entitled to a new purse.

I enjoyed a rare leisurely morning going from shop to shop, looking for just the right purse to contain my new arsenal of supplies. I pricked my finger periodically throughout my travels, and I was happy and relieved to have a steady glucose level. This pump business was working out pretty well.

By the time I got home, it was time for lunch. I had been eating the same thing at the same time every day, much as I had when I was pregnant, to minimize the risk of swings in my glucose level. About an hour after lunch, I pricked my finger. I needed to leave to pick up Emily from school, and I wanted to know my glucose level before I took the thirty-minute, round-trip walk.

I'd spent my first few days on the pump being very nervous before every glucose test, wondering what surprise was in store for me. But I hadn't had any, so I wasn't nervous at all when I pricked my finger after lunch that day. The telltale beep sounded. I looked down at the screen of the PDM and saw a number that shocked me: 397.

I squeezed my eyes closed, trying to remember what to do. I pressed my fingers against my temples, hoping to focus the thoughts in my instantly confused brain. *What did Caryn Hope tell me to do if my glucose level was this high?* Then it came to me: Test for ketones. Right, I needed to test my urine for the presences of ketones. I needed to pee on a ketone test strip.

Ketone test strips are thin, flexible strips about half the length and half the width of a popsicle stick. They have a tiny square area at the bottom of the stick that has to come in contact with urine. You can aim at the tiny square on the stick while you pee, or pee in a cup and dip the square area of the test strip into the pee. Either way, there's bound to be a splash onto your hand. It's impossible to avoid.

Peeing on a stick after you have pricked your finger is, officially, adding insult to injury. The level of ketones is indicated by the color the urine turns the square. A flesh-toned neutral means no ketones. Rosier tones indicate a moderate level. And crimson red means a high level.

I reviewed the package inserts and pulled down my pants, taking care not to dislodge the pod that was now affixed to my belly, sat down on the toilet, and peed onto a test strip. Before I could count to five—the instructions tell you it may take up to fifteen seconds for the results to register—the square end of the test strip had turned an ominous purplish black.

I had so wanted to get through this day without calling Caryn. I wanted my independence back: to feel confident that I could take care of myself without her.

Yet here I was, not knowing what to do. I could feel my pulse in my temples. My heart was racing. I broke into a sweat. I had to call her.

"I'm really high," I told her after she answered the phone, "and I just tested for ketones and got a really high reading on that, too."

"How high was your glucose level?"

I told her.

"Okay, how high on the ketones? More than a trace?"

"Way more. It was the highest level on the color chart. It was practically black."

"So what do you need to do?" she asked. She wanted me to tell her how I was going to troubleshoot this. She wanted me to be self-sufficient, so I could find the right answer on my own the next time something like this happened.

"I need to pick up Emily from school," I answered, missing the point of her question.

"When?"

"In about twenty minutes."

She realized there wasn't time for me to figure this out for myself. "You need to bolus," she said. "I'd say try two units. Test again in an hour. If your pod is working, your glucose level should come down at least 10 percent in the hour. So it should come down about forty points."

"What if it doesn't come down?" I asked.

"If it doesn't come down, call me. We'll need to change your pod. Or you might need to give yourself a shot of insulin." Caryn sounded more serious than I'd heard her before.

"Am I going to be okay for the next hour, when I go to pick up Emily, even though I have all these ketones?"

"You'll be okay for the next hour. But call me if it doesn't come down. And drink lots of water. You need to flush the ketones out. Drink a lot of water and pee a lot."

I drank down a full glass of water, filled a water bottle with more, grabbed my glucose meter, and set out walking to pick Emily up. Her school was about a ten-minute walk through a trail in the woods. I'd been enjoying the walk to school and back every afternoon. It had helped me to get out, to get comfortable doing everyday things as a pumper. I was building confidence every step of the way.

But now things were different. Now I was in a panic the likes of which I hadn't endured in over a decade. The change to the pump was supposed to make my life easier, less scary. It wasn't supposed to make me feel the way I was feeling now. As I walked through the woods, I felt with each step, with each time that I forced myself to put one foot in front of the other, I would break into a thousand messy pieces and end up in a pile on the ground.

The years of worry had taken their toll. I couldn't bear the constant stress anymore. The many bits of me had been strong when they held together, but too many fissures had opened up. It was too much work to hold myself together anymore. I didn't want to be this person with diabetes, this person with a pod stuck to her body, this person with a black-ended ketone test strip in the top of her bathroom wastebasket.

But who will pick up Emily? I thought to myself. *If you break apart into a thousand stupid pieces, who will pick Emily up from school?* That thought, and that thought alone, got me through the woods and to her school. I waited by the flagpole in front for Emily to come out.

"Mommy! You're here!" Emily ran over to greet me.

"Of course I'm here," I answered. "Where else would I be?"

"Why are you upset?" she asked.

"How come you think I'm upset?" I asked. I thought I'd been faking it well. I thought I looked carefree.

"You have that line between your eyes. You always get that when you're upset."

"I'm not upset, sweetie. I'm just squinting. The sun was in my eyes."

"Can we go to the playground?" she asked.

"Not today. We need to go straight home," I told her.

"Why?"

"Well, I'm having a little diabetes problem. I need to go home and call Caryn Hope." My daughter was used to hearing Caryn's name. She was also used to hearing me say I was having a diabetes problem. She'd been hearing that her whole life.

We walked back home. Emily filled me in on every detail of her day. I was feeling stronger with each step, more resolved. I remembered the old days after I was diagnosed, when the panic attacks had set in. I remembered my dear friend Ed telling me I had so much to live for.

This child needs me to be well, I thought. *I need me to be well.* I started to think I could master this pump thing. I could keep fighting the good fight and living my life as an insulin-dependent diabetic. I could play the cards I was dealt. With each step I was a few feet closer to home. A few feet closer to having completed what I thought I couldn't do just a half hour earlier: walking to school and back.

By the time we got home and I got Emily settled, an hour had passed since my last glucose test and my bolus. During that hour, my glucose level should have come down 10 percent, to 350 or so. What with the exercise I got during the walk to school and back, maybe it had come down even more. I stole away into the bathroom, hiding from Emily. She had seen me prick my finger literally thousands of times, but if this one was bad news, I didn't want her to see my reaction.

With the door closed, I pricked my finger, squeezed out the blood, and held it against the test strip. As I waited for the result, I pondered how many hours of my life I've spent waiting for glucose test results, how much time all these chunks of twenty seconds added up to. Before I could run a rough calculation in my mind, the meter beeped, and I looked down: 482. In eleven years and tens of thousands of glucose tests, it was the highest number I'd ever seen. I wasn't getting any insulin from my pod. I might not have had insulin since I changed my pod that morning. I could be heading for DKA.

Quietly I slipped out of the bathroom, grabbed the phone, slipped back into the bathroom and closed the door. I punched in Caryn's cell phone number.

She asked whether my glucose level had gone down.

"No, it's up," I said, the urgency clear in my voice.

"How high?"

"Four hundred eighty-two. That's after bolusing two units an hour ago," I reminded her.

"All right, you're going to need to change your pod."

I groaned loudly. Had Caryn not been able to hear me, I probably would have screamed. Mentally, I was not prepared to change my pod again. I'd done that once already that day, and I'd apparently done it wrong. I wasn't supposed to have to do it again for another three days. Another pod change scared me. Another pod change was another opportunity for me to foul something up.

"Will you stay on the line with me while I change it?" I asked. "I think I know what to do, but I'm just a little freaked out right now."

"Sure, of course I will," she answered.

I set the phone down on the counter and turned on the speaker so that my hands would be free. I needed both hands to deactivate and pull off my old pod, fill a new pod with insulin, and attach it to my body and activate it.

"Amy, before you remove the pod, take a look at it. Can you tell whether there's anything wrong at the infusion site?" The pod had a tiny viewing window at one end, through which you were supposed to be able to see the cannula inserted under your skin. The problem with the viewing window was that it was roughly on the same level as my belly button, and it faced to the outside, which made it very difficult for anyone but a contortionist to look through the window. I gave it my best shot but couldn't see anything.

"Nothing," I reported back to Caryn. Then I tried to gather my thoughts in order to execute my second pod change that day. "Remind me," I said. "Should I be sitting or standing when I put a pod on? I think I was standing this morning when I did it."

"Whatever's most comfortable for you. Either way is fine." *None of this is comfortable for me.*

"I think I'll sit," I said. I closed the lid of the toilet, yanked up my shirt, pulled down the top of my shorts, and sat.

There's a difference in the topography of my abdomen when I'm standing versus sitting. When I'm standing, my abdomen is flat. It's not exactly taut, but it's flat. When I'm sitting, my abdomen becomes a much more challenging terrain, full of peaks and valleys. Rolling hills. I looked at the placement of my pod. When I'd been standing, the pod appeared to fit securely against my abdomen. When I was sitting, however, the pod found itself precariously spanning two hills. The middle of the pod, the part from which the cannula extended, was hovering over a valley. The cannula must have pulled out from under my skin at some point when I had sat down. It had probably become dislodged hours ago when I got into my car to go shopping for my new purse.

I explained my theory to Caryn. "I'm sure that's it," she responded enthusiastically. "Peaks and valleys—I love that. So you need to be sure when you put on a new pod that the cannula's not going to end up in a valley when you sit down or move around."

"Right," I agreed. Having something else to remember each time I changed a pod bore down on me like a weight. I peeled off the old, nonfunctional one, started getting a new one ready to go, and examined my tummy for a new spot to put this one.

As I was doing this, Caryn said, "I'm so glad this is happening now."

"What?" I blurted out.

"It's good that it's happening now, when we're in close contact every day," she said. I winced at the suggestion that Caryn and I wouldn't always be in daily contact. I'd started out this day ready to declare my independence from her, and I found myself now as needy and dependent as ever.

"This is bound to happen to you sometime. And it's going to happen more than once. Now the next time it happens, you'll know just what to do."

I was just beginning to consider her comment when my PDM beeped, signaling that it was ready to tell the new pod to release the needle and insert the tube under my skin. I blinked through the sting of the tube being inserted and then gave myself a bolus of insulin to start to chisel away at my very high glucose level.

"Okay, it's on," I reported. "And I bolused. So now what do I do, wait another hour and test again?"

"You've got it," she said, as if I were an old pro. "You'll be looking for a 10 percent drop in your glucose level in the next hour. And keep drinking water and peeing. It's important to get those ketones out of your system."

"Caryn?" There I was, about to get weepy on her. I can count on one hand the number of times in my life with diabetes that I've found someone who can help me with any aspect of my disease. I can count on one finger the number of times I've had a person available to help me with a crisis at any time, day or night, just by calling her cell phone number. It's always been just me and this relentless disease. Yet for those few weeks I hadn't been alone. Caryn Hope had been with me. She had helped me like no one else had, before or since. "I just want to say thank you. I'll never be able to thank you enough. I don't know what I'll do without you."

"Oh, you'll see, two weeks from now you won't even remember who I am." She was teasing, and I heard the smile in her voice, but she was also laying the groundwork for cutting the cord. She knew she would have to push me out of the nest.

*   *   *

My weaning from Caryn occurred gradually, at my pace. I went back to work a week after I started on the pod. After I was back at work, it was hard to find time for my daily calls with her. We began to communicate by e-mail rather than by phone. Every few days, I'd send her a detailed e-mail with records of my glucose levels, what I'd eaten and when I'd eaten it, how much insulin I'd given myself in the bolus doses, whether and when I'd exercised, how much sleep I'd gotten, and various other factors that might affect my glucose level. She'd e-mail me back with suggestions to help me fine-tune my insulin dosages. Eventually, dozens of e-mails later, Caryn declared me well-regulated, and our communications faded.

Pod changes don't rattle me now. I can change one as easily as when I gave myself shots of insulin. I've changed a pod in the bleachers of a Redskins game, in my office during a conference call, and on a boat in Chesapeake Bay. Give me two minutes, an alcohol swab, a vial of insulin, and a pod, and I'm good to go. That's not to say that I like wearing a pod. Acceptance is not the same thing as contentment.

In fact, I'm basically pissed off about having to use a pump. And I'm pissed off that I have diabetes. Most days of my life I consciously wish that I didn't. But those are the cards I've been dealt.

This hand is what I have to work with. I'd rather wear a pod than not. I'd rather have this little device stuck on me all the time than go back to the regime of multiple injections every day. I'm thankful to be free of the shot.

I saw Dr. Starr a few months after Caryn Hope got me going on the pump. He did my usual blood work, which included my first A1C since I'd been on the pump. He called me with the results a few days later. I didn't hide from his call like I used to. He told me that my A1C was down one full percentage point. In a universe where two or three percentage points can make the difference between developing complications or not, one percentage point is huge. I hung up the phone and shed a few tears of relief, for the first time in way too long. At least for a time, I had regained some level of control over my disease.

31

There's a game Emily likes to play—Ned and Will liked it too when they were young—called "mash." I've never understood why it's called mash, but the game works like this: One person, in this case Emily, writes down on a piece of paper four or five possible choices in four or five different categories. The various categories might be types of clothing or cars or jobs. Paul and I don't see what she writes down. We take turns blindly picking a number between one and five from each category, and then with great delight Emily tells each of us our destiny based on which of her alternatives correspond with the numbers we picked. In a typical game we end up living in an igloo, having rainbow hair and tie-dyed clothes, cleaning toilets as our jobs, with a box on wheels for a car. There's nothing funnier to her than picturing me and Paul in these ridiculous circumstances.

Emily's a kind child, however, and so to make tolerable this existence that she creates for us, she also includes a category for magical powers. So we might get the power to be invisible or to fly or to read minds.

We played mash a while back, while we were on vacation in Maine. We were out to dinner at a restaurant. I'd had a rough hour or so. I'd pricked my finger before leaving the hotel to walk to the restaurant and discovered I was low. I hadn't felt it coming on. But we had reservations and had to get to the restaurant. I chewed down some glucose pills, grabbed a granola bar to eat on the way, and set out with Emily and Paul.

The walk was hard. I was dragging from the low. Things were hazy for me. I couldn't enjoy looking in the shop windows. I couldn't take in the beautiful scenery of the coastal town. I couldn't participate in the conversation. Nothing was registering. I let Paul and Emily walk a bit ahead, so she wouldn't have to worry about my vacancy.

When we got to the restaurant, I immediately gobbled down some bread, wanting to get more carbs into my system. I was starting to feel better, and the outing was becoming fun for me at last. I was part of the experience now, not partially absent.

When our dinner eventually came, I pricked my finger so I'd know how much insulin to bolus before I ate. "Ugh," I groaned when I saw my number. I usually try not to groan in front of Emily, but I was just so damn frustrated. Now I was high. Over 200. There was just no winning.

"Are you low again, Mommy?"

"No, I'm high now. But it's okay. I'll be fine after dinner." I said it with confidence, as though I believed it in the hope that she would. I hated how it worried her.

"Want to play mash?" she asked. Paul and I made our blind selections in the game. Emily announced Paul's outcome first. "You live in a hut, you drive a Volkswagen hippie van, you have a pet rat, and your job is coach of the Redskins. But guess what your magical power is?"

"I don't know, sweets. If I'm the coach of the Redskins I'm going to need some kind of magic."

"Listen. Here's your magical power..." Emily looked over at me, smiling, her eyes shining. "You have the power to make Type 1 diabetes go away."

"Wow," Paul and I said. "What an awesome power that would be."

Then it was my turn to pick the numbers that would determine my fate. I intentionally picked different numbers than Paul had in each category because I wanted to have a different outcome. I wanted to give her a different set of circumstances to laugh at. So I was surprised when the results were revealed, to learn that my magical power was also the power to make Type 1 diabetes go away.

"Hey, wait a minute," I said. "It's a great power, but how did we both get it? I picked a different number than Daddy."

"You just did."

"Let me see your paper, honey." She resisted. "Come on, hand it over." Looking me in the eyes, she handed it over. There, in her most careful third-grade hand, under the heading Magical Powers, were the following five options:

1. The power to make Diabetes Type 1 go away.
2. The power to make Diabetes Type 1 go away.
3. The power to make Diabetes Type 1 go away.
4. The power to make Diabetes Type 1 go away.
5. The power to make Diabetes Type 1 go away.

"Sweetie," I said, my eyes dampening. "You're an amazing person. You're really something."

"Does anyone have that power, Mommy? I mean, for real? The power to make it go away?"

"I think someone does. Yes, I'm sure someone does."

"But why haven't they done it?"

"Well, it's like the scientific method that you studied in class. They have to have a hypothesis, and they have to go through lots of steps, and if it doesn't work right at the end, then they have to go back to the beginning and start all over again. So it takes a long time. But they're working on it."

She paused to consider my answer and then asked, "When they figure it out, will you have to wear a pod anymore?"

"Nope, I won't."

"Will you have to prick your finger anymore?"

"Nope, I won't have to do that, either."

"Not ever? Not once?"

"Maybe once. Maybe I'd have to go to my doctor once a year, and he'd prick my finger and tell me I still don't have diabetes."

The three of us were quiet for a while as we each wondered whether that's a life I'll ever know. Emily broke the silence.

"It's going to be great when that happens, Mommy."

"It *is* going to be great, honey. It sure is."

32

I got onto the subway feeling that I'd been through a battle. I didn't even really feel like crying, as I sometimes do, because I was too far gone for that. I just wanted it all to stop. *For the love of God, can't this just stop?* The diabetes was enough. Honestly, it was more than enough. I couldn't bear a complication.

I wondered what I looked like to other people as I got on the subway. At first glance I probably looked like a well-dressed, middle-aged woman. Slightly tired perhaps, could stand to lose a few pounds maybe, but really no worse for the wear. I had on a pencil skirt that was actually flattering, a sleeveless top with a nice jacket over it, and very appropriate accessories. I was having a good hair day, and I had a nice handbag. So why did I close my eyes sharply and draw in my breath as I sat down? Why did I wince when accidentally, out of habit, I put my heavy purse in my lap? Why, if they really looked closely, did I have a slight lump on my left thigh that showed through the skirt when I sat down? And what was that one accessory that so clearly did not match my perfectly professional persona? The large white plastic bag labeled, of all things, "Patient Supplies, Room 651a."

What no one would have guessed, what only I knew, was that beneath the brown skirt, beneath the polished exterior, was an open wound in my left thigh that I likened to a bullet hole. A bullet hole with a wide tail of ribbon dangling out of it, all covered with a doubled-over, taped-on square of gauze. Sure, I'm prone to hyperbole. But the only way for me to gird myself for the next few weeks was to think of it as a bullet hole. That's the only type of wound I had ever associated with packing.

*   *   *

I considered myself lucky that in five and a half years of being on an insulin pump, I'd never gotten an infection at my pump infusion site. The infusion site is the place on my body where a needle inserts a cannula, a tube, under my skin for a steady stream of insulin to be dispensed around the clock. The needle retracts after the tube is inserted. It's common to get infections at an infusion site, either from irritation to the skin caused by the adhesive that holds the pump in place or from bacteria introduced when the needle inserts the tube under the skin.

Infections are a scary thing for a person with diabetes. We have compromised immune systems that don't fight infections well. We experience worse outcomes from infections than people who don't have diabetes. In a best-case scenario, we heal more slowly and require longer hospitalizations. In a worst-case scenario, bacteria from an infection can spread to the bloodstream, potentially creating a lethal condition known as bacteremia. An infection around a toenail or a blister gone bad on a foot can lead to amputation if the infection can't be stopped. So I was grateful not to ever have had an infection on or under my skin.

When I remove my insulin pod every three days to discard it and get a new one going on a new site on my body, I usually have some mild irritation. Often I have a raised mark—the size of a small bug bite—where the cannula has been under my skin. Sometimes I have a colorful bruise, an elliptical shape in brilliant purples and reds. Other times, there's a small hematoma, a bubble of blood around where the cannula has been. And always there's a patch of itchy, irritated, red skin, a patch larger than the pod itself, where the adhesive sat.

Sure, all of this was bothersome. But could I deal with it? Yes. This was nothing. The raised mark would go down, the bruise would fade, the hematoma would flatten out, and the skin irritation could be remedied with a good dose of hydrocortisone cream. It was nothing that would slow me down before activating a new pod on another spot on my arm or on my abdomen or on my thigh, to face the same outcomes when I'd change that one three days later.

I like to wear my insulin pod on my thigh in the summertime, with "like" being a relative term in this context. I don't like to have it on my arm because I don't want it to show if I wear a short-sleeved or sleeveless shirt or dress. I never like to have it on my abdomen, even though it is quite effective there, because I don't need extra inches and a lump there. So I've found that the front of my thigh, slightly toward the inside, where it's a little fleshier, is a good place. It works with my clothes. It works and is nearly undetectable when I wear shorts and even when I'm in a skirted bathing suit. It works for sleeping with my husband. It just works well there. Usually.

Sometimes I can barely feel my pod. I put it on, and then later I have to pat around on my body to remember where it is. Those are the good days. When I find it, I drum on it lightly with my finger-nails and think, *Ah, thank you for being such a good pod that I didn't even remember where you were. Thank you for not hurting me.*

But sometimes my pod does hurt. Sometimes the initial sting of the needle inserting the cannula is surprisingly sharp, and the pain dulls but doesn't quite go away. Sometimes the adhesive is not quite right, and it pinches my skin or pulls uncomfortably, and I then have to decide whether I can deal with the discomfort for the next few days or whether I should change the pod. Changing the pod means wasting insulin. And if I've just filled a pod with insulin, I can't stand to throw it away.

I can never have enough insulin in reserve, though my prescription plan seems committed to ensuring that I can't be too comfortable. For instance, I used to be able to get two vials at a time, and now I can get only one. At any one time I probably have three or four vials with a tiny bit of insulin left, some maybe half full. But there's nothing like the assurance of having a couple of unopened vials in the fridge. It's better than money in the bank.

The vials are glass. If a vial drops, it's gone. To shatter a vial of insulin is to instantly give your house the unmistakable scent of an emergency room. It was so surprising to me the first time it happened. The scent spread so quickly. It was amazing that such a powerful and distinctive aroma could come from such a tiny vial. Insulin also loses its effectiveness if it isn't kept within a narrow, relatively cool temperature range. Insulin in a purse, briefcase, or backpack is in danger of becoming overheated and impotent if it isn't kept cool enough. Shattering a vial of insulin or realizing I have left the insulin in my purse in a hot car for two hours on a summer day gives me a suffocating sense of panic. *That was my last full vial. Can I get more? Will the pharmacist believe me?* It's crazy to have a little vial of clear fluid on which my life depends. It's even crazier that I would have to beg for leniency from the insurance company if my reserve becomes diminished too soon.

The pod that I'd had on my left thigh had been uncomfortable from the moment I'd activated it, but stubbornly, I didn't take it off. I didn't want to waste the insulin. It was from a fresh, new vial. Being familiar with all sorts of discomfort the pod might cause, I thought this one was an adhesive discomfort. It was mild, nothing that kept me awake at night, but certainly noticeable enough that I didn't have to go patting around for the pod. I knew right where this one was, because I could feel it all the time. I left it on for three days.

When at last it was time to remove the pod, I was so relieved. I couldn't wait to peel it off, rub on the hydrocortisone cream to calm my inflamed skin, and move the next pod onto new terrain. The irritated skin was angrier than usual and felt tightly drawn and slightly warm. But I kept moving. I had a new pod to put on, this time on my abdomen. And I had things to do. It was a work day, just like any other, and I couldn't slow down because of a painful spot on my leg.

Paul and I found ourselves childless that evening, and so we met for dinner: he on his way home from work and I joining him from my home office. I'd been wearing baggy gym shorts all day in my home office, and for dinner I changed into a pair of snug jeans. I try not to complain. But when I sat down at the table with Paul, I nearly cried out when the fabric of my jeans pulled tightly against the patch on my thigh.

"God, that hurts," I said, closing my eyes.

"What does?"

"Where I took my pod off today. It's killing me. It's never felt like this." I laid my hand gently over the spot that hurt. "It's hot, too. I can feel it through my jeans. If it's not better in the morning, I'm going to urgent care."

The next morning, Saturday, the angry patch was still there and still hot to the touch. There was also a little lump in the middle of it, about the size of a small pea. It hurt like crazy. Paul was out on an early-morning bike ride, and I waited for him to get home so I could leave Emily with him. I was dressed and ready to go. As soon as he walked in the door, I grabbed my purse and said casually, trying not to alarm Emily, "I'm going out for a bit. I should be home in a few hours."

That was the wrong approach. I never breeze out the door and say I'll be back in a few hours. If I'm gone for more than ninety minutes, the household nearly breaks down. "What? Where are you going?" Paul and Emily asked.

"Nowhere, just some errands."

"Errands? What errands? I didn't know you were doing errands today."

There was no evading them. "Okay, I'm going to urgent care. The place on my leg is really bad. I think it's infected. I want to see if I need antibiotics."

"Can't you go on Monday?" Paul asked. "It's such a pretty day. I was thinking maybe we could do something outside."

I flew off the handle. "You think I have time to go to the doctor on Monday? Did you forget I have a job and I have to go work on Monday? Did you forget I have to pick up the dry cleaning on Monday and go to the grocery store if we want to have any food to eat next week? And pick up Emily and cook dinner and do the laundry and walk the dog? So no, I don't have time to go to the doctor on Monday.

"And oh, by the way," I continued, "I don't care that it's a beautiful day. I'd rather sit in the waiting room of a stinking urgent care office on Route 1 while my thigh is throbbing and I'm scared to death that I have an infection. That's what I want to do on this beautiful day."

"Um, Mom," Emily asked hesitantly. "Are you okay?"

"I'm fine, Emily," I said testily. Then I closed the door loudly and stormed off. I didn't make it far, though, before I turned turn around, went back into the house, and inflicted a little more fury on Paul. I wasn't going to be the only one who suffered today. "What do you not understand about this, Paul?" I yelled at him. "I have an infection. In my leg. I can't let that wait until Monday. What don't you get about this?" And then I stormed off again.

The admitting nurse at the urgent care facility took my medical history and asked me to explain the condition that brought me in. When I explained that the trouble spot was at the site of my last insulin pump infusion site, she said, "So you're Type 1?" She knew what she was talking about. She knew who I was. Unfortunately the doctor who came in after her was not so well informed.

She took one look at the patch on my thigh and said, "It's infected. But I can't get your insulin pump out of there, so you're going to have to go to the emergency room."

"What? I don't get what you're saying. My insulin pump is not in there."

"Well, what's under there?" She meant what was under my skin, causing the lump and the irritation.

"Nothing's under there. I mean, I think there's an infection under there. But there's no pump under there."

"Insulin pumps are implanted under the skin, and you're going to need to have it surgically removed," she informed me.

Get me out of here, I thought.

I showed her where my new pod was, on my stomach. "The irritation is where my old pump was before I moved it."

"I don't know anything about what insulin pumps are like today," she said without a trace of irony. A licensed physician, the lone doctor seeing emergency patients during weekends and off hours, didn't know how an insulin pump made in this century functions.

I was beyond annoyed with her, and I felt like walking out, but I needed to get a prescription for an antibiotic. "Oh, I'm sure it's hard to keep up with the technology," I said lightly, as if it were completely understandable that she missed twenty-five years' worth of advancements in the treatment of diabetes. "Do you think I should be on antibiotics if it's infected?"

"I do. I'm going to put you on Cipro."

I thought Cipro sounded odd. The only time I'd heard of Cipro before was in the post-9/11 anthrax scare. But I assumed if Cipro could beat anthrax, it would work on anything.

*   *   *

"Why'd she put you on Cipro?" Dr. Starr, my endocrinologist, asked when I called him first thing Monday morning. The place on my leg was no better. It was worse. The small pea had expanded into a grape. It hurt like hell. It was red and tight and warm to the touch.

"I have no idea. That's just what she told me to take."

"Cipro doesn't kill the type of bacteria this would be. This is probably staph. This is bacteria in tissue. Cipro doesn't get that."

"So what should I be taking?"

"I'll call something in that works on staph. Do you have a fever?"

"No." I'd been checking my temperature twice a day.

"Then take the new antibiotic for two days, see if it gets better, and call me if it doesn't."

Two days later nothing had changed, except the grape had swollen into a golf ball. I could barely stand to have the weight of a piece of fabric on it. Sitting and standing were painful, as the skin stretched to accommodate the golf ball. I called the doctor, who told me to come to his office.

Finally, I'm going to see someone who will to do something right.

Dr. Starr took one look at my thigh and said, "Oh, this doesn't look good. This is a bad infection. It looks like an abscess. I'm going to need to send you to a surgeon."

"A surgeon? Why?"

"I can't drain an abscess here." He touched the swollen lump, pressing gently around the edges to get a feel for how big it was, for where its boundaries were. He considered it a bit longer and then said, "Well, I could try, I guess, if you want me to."

"Oh yes, I want you to try. Please try." I was, happy, excited in fact, that my favorite doctor might be able to drain my abscess. Now that I knew it was an abscess, I didn't want to go to a surgeon.

I lay on the examining table as he inserted a needle into the lump and drew some fluid out. It was incredibly painful. I tried not to cry out. In my silence, tears streamed out of the outside corners of my eyes. In all my years of seeing Dr. Starr, I had never cried in front of him. He saw the tears spilling.

"I'm sorry, Mrs. Ryan." He still called me Mrs. Ryan after all these years. "Am I hurting you?"

"It does hurt," I said, exhaling deeply. I had been holding my breath. "But it's okay."

"Do you want me to stop?"

"No, keep trying. I'm all right."

He tried a bit more, each new attempt more painful than the last. "I can't get it. I can't get all the pus out."

"Okay. You can stop." I wanted it out. I wanted my leg not to hurt anymore. I wanted the infection to be sucked out. I would go to the surgeon.

For a person with Type 1 diabetes, an infection is a thing to be feared. An infection in a limb inspires a fear worse than dread.

Although I don't go around searching for amputation stories, I didn't think I'd ever heard of a leg amputation resulting from an infection. Toe amputations, foot amputations, below-the-knee amputations, sure. In my mind, though, a leg was not too far of a stretch. If a toe infection went too far, it could lead to a foot amputation. If a foot infection went too far, it could lead to a below-the-knee amputation. What had started as a small, pea-sized infection in my thigh had grown quickly into an infected golf ball. What if it grew into a baseball? *This is how things spin out of control*, I thought. *This is how it starts.*

I found my way into the surgery clinic at the university hospital. I filled out the paperwork and handed it to the receptionist.

She accepted the clipboard with my forms on it and asked, "Do you have a loved one?"

"A what?"

"A loved one—a friend or a family member."

"Oh, I do. I have lots of loved ones. I have the most wonderful loved ones..." I trailed off dreamily. It made me momentarily happy to think of them all.

"Mrs. Ryan," she said, looking up at me over the glasses that were perched on the end of her nose. "Do you have any loved ones here today?" She looked at me as if I were the most simpleminded person she had encountered in quite some time.

"Oh, I see what you're asking. No, I don't have any loved ones here today."

"You're alone?"

"Yes, I'm alone." *At the bottom of it all, I am so often alone.*

"You can put your belongings in this," she said, handing me a large plastic bag.

A nurse led me into the procedure room, took my vital signs, and gave me a giant pair of paper bloomers to put on. They were sized to fit a sumo wrestler, with elastic around the waist and the bottom of each leg. Kind of like a giant diaper cover. At least I could keep my underwear on beneath and my shirt up top while the surgeon did whatever it was he was going to do to the raging lump in my thigh. I still wasn't quite sure what that was going to be.

The nurse left the room. Next in was a medical student. I was at a teaching hospital. If I had to be at a hospital, I was glad it was a university hospital. Having students around reminded me of the hospital where my mother had practiced as a nurse. The boy who came in—I have to call him a boy even though he was probably in his late twenties—was studying to be a surgeon. He was kind, thorough, curious, intelligent, and courteous—everything a patient would want a doctor to be. I wished his parents could see him with me, how thoughtful and caring he was. They would be so proud. He reminded me of my older stepson, Ned.

The student left the room, and the surgeon came in and introduced himself, with the student at his side. "Mrs. Ryan, let's see," he said, looking at my chart. "So you have Type 1 diabetes, and you wear an insulin pump. You have an underactive thyroid, and you have rheumatoid arthritis."

"That's me."

"So you're a healthy woman."

"Right," I said bitterly.

"No, you are," he said. "I can tell by looking at you. You look healthy. You look like you take care of yourself. Lots of people with your list don't look so good."

"Well, thanks. I try." He was easy to talk to, and I thought that if I could just keep our conversation going, maybe he would forget that he was about to do something that was going to hurt me. But he knew why he was there.

I lay on the procedure table. The surgeon told me he was going to give me an injection of a local anesthetic, and the injection would sting and hurt. But after that, I shouldn't feel anything. If I did feel anything, I should let him know, and he would give me another injection of the anesthetic. He was going to use a scalpel to open the abscess, and then he would drain the pus out. When he was finished, he'd leave it open, and we'd have to pack the wound. That didn't make much sense to me. I didn't know how you could leave something like that open, and I didn't know what "pack" meant.

He gave me the first injection, and I felt the searing pain of the needle going into the infected mass. The burning subsided, and he asked if I could feel him pressing on my lump with the scalpel. I could tell that there was pressure, but the scalpel didn't hurt.

He worked for a while at whatever he was doing, extracting with a needle, scraping with something. "There's a lot in here," he said. "And it's deep. It's deeper than I thought. How deep does the needle of your insulin pump go?"

"I don't know. I don't see the needle. It retracts before I ever see it. I only see the cannula."

"How deep does that go?"

I held up my thumb and index finger.

"That's why it's so deep, I think. The needle pushed it way down in there." He moved to a slightly new area and was just starting to say, "Can you feel that?" when I screamed in pain. "Okay, there are a few pockets here. I'm going to give you a little more anesthesia; then you won't feel a thing."

He continued in this way for a while, getting what he could, probing a new area until I felt it, and then giving me another injection of the anesthetic. When at last he was finished, I was feeling no pain. "I think I got it all," he said. "Mrs. Ryan, I want you to sit up here, and I'm going to show you what I did and how you're going to pack it."

When I was lying down, I hadn't been able to see what he was doing. The billowing bloomers were so puffed out that they obscured my view. When I sat up, however, I could see right away what he had done. It looked as if he had drilled a hole in my thigh. There was a hole, an actual hole, about the circumference of my little finger on my left thigh. I couldn't tell how deep it was, but it was well beyond superficial.

"Oh my God," I said, and lay back down. I'm not squeamish, but this rocked me. This wasn't like anything I'd ever seen or imagined. I've never fainted. I've never felt like I was going to faint—until I saw the hole in my leg.

"Are you okay, Mrs. Ryan?"

"I don't know. I can't look at that. That's crazy."

"Well, we need to have you look one more time because we need to show you how to pack it."

I raised up on my elbows, so I could see what he was doing while still supporting myself. He had a long wooden stick, like a giant Q-tip without cotton on one end. And he had a canister of something called packing material, which looked similar to the curling ribbon that I used to decorate presents at birthdays and Christmas. He took one end of the ribbon, pressed the stick against it, and then pushed it into the hole. Then with the stick, as if he were doing needlepoint, he made a neat accordion pleat and pushed in another fold of the ribbon. And so on, until inches of the pleated material had been packed into the hole.

I couldn't believe what I was seeing. The image that came into my mind was of an autopsy scene in *CSI*: The medical examiner does something to a corpse that should cause it to cry out in pain, like inserting tweezers under a fingernail. I was watching the surgeon pack a ribbon into an anesthetized hole in my leg with a stick, and I couldn't feel a thing. That was so wrong. You're not supposed to be able to poke a stick way down into your leg. When he had packed in as much as the hole would accept, he left a little tail hanging out. He covered the whole mess with large gauze pad and secured the edges with surgical tape.

"We do it this way. We leave it open because it needs to heal from the inside out. You don't want the skin to close over it. That'd trap the pus inside, and you'd find yourself back in here doing this again. So it has to stay open and drain. Now tomorrow," he continued, "you're going to grab the tail that's hanging out, pull the packing out, wash the opening with soap and water, and pack it again."

I didn't hesitate a moment before I said, "I really don't think I can do that."

"You can do it. You want this to get better, right? You don't want me to have to open it up again, do you? So you're going to do this for two weeks, and then you're going to come back in and see me."

"Two weeks?" I asked feebly.

"Two weeks. And we'll see how it looks then. Now the anesthesia is going to start wearing off, and you're going to feel some pain. I'm writing you a prescription for Tylenol with codeine. Take it if you need it. You don't have to feel the pain."

A smiling nurse came into the room with another big, white plastic bag.

She handed me the bag, and I looked inside. There were several packs of gauze pads, canisters of the packing material, surgical tape, and the long sticks that I would need to pack the hole. I accepted the bag and was left alone in the room. I took off the bloomers, put on my skirt, holding my breath as it passed over the gauze-wrapped spot on my thigh. I hobbled out of the surgery suite, stopping in the ladies' room to prick my finger. I had to know what my glucose level was for the long journey home. I was still a painful walk, a short subway ride, and a drive in rush-hour traffic away from my actual loved ones.

*   *   *

I awoke at around 4:00 a.m. with a searing pain in my thigh. It felt like it was being gouged with a hot poker. I got up, went into the bathroom, and took a couple of ibuprofen. I hadn't gotten my prescription for the Tylenol with codeine filled. I figured it was not a good time for me to get hooked on a narcotic. I needed to use the bathroom, and when I did, I saw that the gauze that was covering my hole was soaked in blood. I hadn't noticed at first, but my pajama shorts had blood on them, too, over the spot where the hole was. I needed to change the gauze. That's what the doctor had said: If there's blood coming through the gauze, then change it.

I turned on a brighter light in the bathroom. I was wide awake now. I closed the toilet lid and sat down. I wondered if there was a way I could change the gauze that wouldn't require me to see the hole. But there was no way around it. I removed the tape around the gauze carefully and then lifted the gauze. I gasped at what I saw. The tail of the ribbon that was coming out of the hole was black and hard, matted against the skin around the hole and caked in dried blood. The edges of the hole were purplish red, inflamed, and swollen. I didn't let myself look at it for more than few seconds.

I covered it with a new gauze pad, put on some clean pajama bottoms, and went to back to bed. I couldn't cuddle with Paul because I couldn't bear the pressure of his body against my wound. I lay awake, wondering how in God's name I was going to pull that ribbon out of the hole the next day.

When I got out of bed for the day a few hours later, there was blood on my pajama shorts again, and blood on the sheets. I hobbled around the house, getting Emily off to school. The edges of the hole pulled and hurt when I walked, when I bent over, and when I moved from sitting to standing, or vice versa.

After Emily was on the bus, I went into the bathroom to do what I had to do: Pull the packing material out, take a shower, wash the hole with soap and water, and then repack it. I sat on the toilet lid as I had done a few hours earlier. I gently lifted a corner of the gauze and peered under it. I closed it back up. I felt as lightheaded as I had the day before in the procedure room. I needed to have someone there with me, outside the door, to get help if I keeled over.

I called my sister-in-law, Tania, the one who had hosted the dinner party that I'd attended so many years before, right after my diagnosis, when my glucose meter was like a new toy. I told her what had happened and what I had to do. She said she'd be right over.

I asked her to wait outside the bathroom and listen for the sound of my head hitting the floor. I was only half kidding.

I sat down on the toilet lid again. I lifted the gauze again and groaned out loud when I saw the caked-on mess of dried blood.

"Amy, are you okay?" she asked from outside the door.

"It's so bad, Tania. I don't know how I'm going to do it."

"I'm coming in," she said. "Can I come in?"

"Sure, come in."

"Eww, wow," she said when she saw it. "Eww."

"I know." I used my fingernail to work the tail of the ribbon off of the spot where it was stuck to my skin. I gave it a little tug, and one pleat of the ribbon pulled out. "Oh my God, oh my God, oh my God." It had burned like hell getting that one little notch to come out.

"Does it hurt?"

"Oh man, it hurts." I continued pulling the ribbon gently, with each fold of the ribbon tugging and burning inside the hole before it popped loose and emerged. We were amazed at how long the ribbon was. It was probably five inches. Not that the hole was five inches deep, but because the ribbon had been folded so many times—to pack as much in as possible.

Tania took the bloody, pus-soaked ribbon out of my hand, wrapped it in toilet paper, and threw it in the trashcan. She started the shower for me. I stood up to move toward the shower, and a thick stream of fluid, resembling motor oil more than blood, spilled out of the hole and rushed down my leg, spreading over my foot and onto the floor. I bent to try to mop it up, and yelped in pain when I tried to bend over. I caught a glimpse of myself in the mirror, naked, an insulin pump on my abdomen, blood pouring from the hole in my leg. *Good God, is that me? How is that me?*

"You get in the shower. I'll get it," Tania said, grabbing more toilet paper to clean up the mess on the floor.

I stepped carefully into the shower and let the water run over me. I enjoyed about two seconds of the calming sensation before the water washed over the hole. It felt like someone had pushed in a lit match. The burning subsided after a while. I washed the opening with soap and water, cringing when my hand moved over its tight, swollen edges. I stayed in the shower as long as I could. I didn't want to do what I had to do when I got out.

When at last I turned off the water and emerged from the shower, I saw that Tania had set up a nice little procedure area for me. She had put a clean towel over the toilet lid so I wouldn't be sitting on the cold porcelain. She had moved my surgical supplies out of the generic plastic hospital bag and into a pretty shopping bag with grosgrain ribbon handles. She had laid out a clean washcloth on which rested a packing stick, the packing material, a small pair of scissors, a gauze pad, and surgical tape. She had brought me two glasses of water—one still and one sparkling—because she wasn't sure which I would prefer.

"Tania," I said. "Look what you did."

I dried off and sat on the towel-covered toilet lid. I looked at the hole. The blood had stopped spilling out after I got in the shower. All it needed now was a good few inches of packing material. I cut off a length of the ribbon and laid one end atop the hole. I eased the stick onto it and tried to poke it down into the hole. It hurt terribly. "I can't do this, Tania. I can't do it. I can't do it. I can't do it." She watched me with her brow furrowed, a pained expression on her face. It was not pretty to watch what I was doing.

But each time I said I couldn't do it, I made another fold and pushed a little more of the packing ribbon into the hole. I would get it done in spite of myself, in spite of the fact that I didn't think I could.

When at last I could get no more packing into the hole, I cut the ribbon and left a tail hanging out. I covered it with a fresh white square of gauze. Then I mopped the sweat off my face and stomach. I had been sweating bullets.

I didn't have to look at the hole until tomorrow, but I couldn't stop thinking about it. I couldn't stop thinking, *This is how it starts. It starts with an infection.* And now I had an open wound on my body—an open wound that could become contaminated. The skillful surgeon had sucked out the pus and carved out the infected tissue, but there was all that fresh red tissue with a big opening to welcome new contaminants. There was a ripe spot calling out for a germ of bacteria to nestle into the hole and then maybe spread to my bloodstream. How was I going to keep that thing open for two weeks and not get another infection?

I needed another loved one. This time it was Delia. From the moment she and I had met, it was if we had known each other our whole lives. Few people cheer me up like she does. Delia knows lots of people who have diabetes. She knows lots of war stories, and she knows a lot of success stories. I wanted to hear a success story. I wanted to know if she had ever encountered what was happening to me. I wanted her to tell me that it happens all the time, and it always comes out fine.

"Oh, my gosh, you poor thing," she said when I told her about the abscess. "I'm so sorry you're going through this. But no, I've never heard about anything like that."

"Delia, I'm afraid this is how it starts. You know, it starts with an infection." She knew exactly what I meant.

"You're not going to get another infection, Amy," she said. "The doctor got it out. And you're on antibiotics. You're going to keep it clean, and it's going to be fine. It is."

"But two weeks, Delia. Two weeks with an open wound in my leg. And it could be longer than that if it doesn't heal right."

"Listen, Amy," she said. "I don't want you to think I'm comparing, because I'd never compare what you're going through to someone else."

Then Delia told me about a woman she knew. She was younger than I was, but she had survived with Type 1 diabetes for thirty years. Just a few days earlier, she had told Delia she felt as if she had spiders running up and down her lower leg. The first time she noticed it, she brushed her leg to knock them off.

"But they weren't there, Amy," Delia said.

"God, no," I said with horror.

Her friend was developing neuropathy, nerve damage to her lower extremities that could make her feel like bugs were on her skin, that eventually could make her feel like bees were stinging her, and that ultimately could result in loss of all feeling in that area. A loss of feeling is a typical precursor to an infection that can lead to amputation. A blister that goes undetected on a foot can quickly spiral out of control.

"Her doctor told her it may not be reversible," Delia said. Then she was quiet for a moment. "But yours *is* reversible, Amy. You caught it in time. Yours is going to get better. It sucks, and it hurts, and I wish you didn't have to go through this, but yours is going to get better. Just watch."

Maybe Delia was right. Maybe this would get better. I had my bullet hole to take care of, but maybe in the end it would turn out that, at least this time, I'd dodged the real bullet.

33

The hole in my leg gradually filled in. It took longer than I expected. For two full months I unpacked, cleaned, repacked, and carefully covered that hole every day. It was discouraging in the beginning, when I couldn't discern much of a change on a daily basis. But then one day, I pulled out the packing to find that the edges were no longer purplish red. They were pink. A few days later the edges were nearly my normal skin color. And a few days after that, I could tell for the first time that the hole was a little less deep because it wouldn't accept as much packing tape as the day before. It was beginning to repair itself.

I became strangely fascinated with the hole—with watching it heal. I began not to mind it so much. I almost began to like it because I could see it getting better. I didn't wonder, as with so many things in my life, whether it would get better or when it would get better. I could actually see it getting better. Every single day. It was an amazing thing to watch.

So many things make holes in our lives. Unexpected, frightening events that change your life forever can come out of nowhere. They can leave you with a raw opening somewhere so deep within yourself that you don't know how or whether or when it might fill in. All you know is that you have some new space that you didn't have yesterday and that your life is different now.

Holes have opened up in my life before—gaping ones that justify hyperbole. When I was diagnosed with diabetes, I could almost physically feel the abyss it created—the deep pit of fear, anger, uncertainty, and sadness. But somehow, over time, while I didn't even know it was happening, that abyss filled in. I can look at my life, I can look at who I am, and I can feel that the huge hole that diabetes bored into me has healed and closed now.

So many things have flowed in to fill the void: A husband who loves me more today than he did the day before my diagnosis; two stepsons whom I've had the privilege of seeing into young adulthood (sure, there were new spaces in my life when they moved on to college and beyond, but those were filled over time with the new pleasure of knowing them as adults); a thirteen-year-old daughter I thought I might never have, who is a source of joy every day of my life; a sister who is cancer-free and going strong nearly nine years after her breast cancer; and friends who can make me laugh until my stomach aches, even in the darkest of times.

I'm not going to turn this into a happy, facile ending. I'm not going to diminish the struggle with a cliché and swear that diabetes suddenly made me aware, for the very first time, of those things that are truly important in my life. But I don't want to give short shrift to gratitude, and I also want to offer some hard-won advice: Holes are going to appear in your life. There's no predicting them, and there's no stopping them. The trouble with them is not just that they happen, but that they seem to take forever to heal, if they heal at all. Some may not. But when they do, you can't always feel them filling in or know when they will be better until they are. The answer is in believing that they can.

Acknowledgements

I would like to thank Nina Sichel for helping me to find my story and for reviewing and providing editorial support on an early version of the manuscript. Were it not for Nina, I wouldn't have known I had a story to tell.

I am grateful to my friend and colleague Anthony Franze for pushing me, even when he knew I didn't want to hear it, and for not letting me let this project die. Anthony gives new meaning to the words "constant encouragement."

Thanks to my friends who read early drafts of the manuscript and encouraged me to pursue this project—Janet Hamlin, Ida Bostian, Kristina Heiberger, Delia Whitfield, Larry Soler, Aaron Kowalski, Christine Kirk, and Ann Stanley.

I will be forever indebted to Sue Petrie and Bill Patrick for taking an interest in my story and devoting themselves to this book. Sue, thanks for writing "don't stress about this" in just about every e-mail you ever sent me. Bill, thanks for your patient, thorough, thoughtful, and personal editing, and your endless good humor, particularly at a time when things weren't easy in your life.

To my mother, sister, and brother, who have always supported me in whatever I do, and my late father, whom I know would be proud.

Most of all, I thank my family; Paul, Ned, Will, and Emily. Thank you for putting up with me. Thank you for believing in me. Thank you for being there for all the highs, all the lows, and those rare days when we can almost forget I have diabetes. Without you, this story would have no meaning. You are everything. Moku say.

About Hudson Whitman

Hudson Whitman is a new small press affiliated with Excelsior College in upstate New York.

Our tagline is "Books That Make a Difference," and we aim to publish high-quality nonfiction books and multimedia projects in areas that complement Excelsior's academic strengths: education, nursing, health care, military interests, business and technology, with one "open" category, American culture and society.

If you would like to submit a manuscript or proposal, please review the guidelines on our website, hudsonwhitman.com. Feel free to send a note with any questions. We endeavor to respond as soon as possible.

OTHER TITLES BY HUDSON WHITMAN

The Language of Men
Anthony D'Aries (print and e-book)

Courageous Learning:
Finding a New Path through Higher Education
John Ebersole and William Patrick (print and e-book)

Saving Troy:
A Year with Firefighters and Paramedics in a Battered City
William Patrick (e-book only)

CPSIA information can be obtained at www.ICGtesting.com
Printed in the USA
LVOW130404120413

328860LV00001B/37/P